Cytopathology
and Bone Lesi

MW00843307

For further volumes, go to
http://www.springer.com/series/6996

Walid E. Khalbuss, MD, PhD, FIAC

University of Pittsburgh Medical Center, Shadyside Hospital,
Pittsburgh, PA, USA

Anil V. Parwani, MD, PhD

University of Pittsburgh Medical Center, Shadyside Hospital,
Pittsburgh, PA, USA

Cytopathology of Soft Tissue and Bone Lesions

Including Chapters 6 & 7 Co-authored by:
Živa Pohar-Marinšek, MD, PhD
Institute of Oncology, Ljubljana, Slovenia, EU
and Chapters 8 & 9 Co-authored by:
Marilyn M. Bui, MD, PhD
Moffitt Cancer Center, Tampa, FL, USA

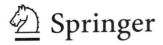

Springer

Walid E. Khalbuss, M.D., Ph.D.
University of Pittsburgh
Medical Center
Shadyside Hospital
Pittsburgh, PA, USA

Anil V. Parwani, M.D., Ph.D.
University of Pittsburgh
Medical Center
Shadyside Hospital
Pittsburgh, PA, USA

ISBN 978-1-4419-6498-4   e-ISBN 978-1-4419-6499-1
DOI 10.1007/978-1-4419-6499-1
Springer New York Dordrecht Heidelberg London

Library of Congress Control Number: 2010930606

Printed on acid-free paper

Springer is part of Springer Science+Business Media (www.springer.com)

To my family:
Mother (Fatimah); Wife (Hanah); and My Kids (Feras, Sarah, &
Zach).

Walid E. Khalbuss, MD, PhD, FIAC

To my parents, my wife and my children.

Anil V. Parwani, MD, PhD

Series Preface

The subspeciality of cytopathology is 60 years old and has become established as a solid and reliable discipline in medicine. As expected, cytopathology literature has expanded in a remarkably short period of time, from a few textbooks prior to the 1980s to a current and substantial library of texts and journals devoted exclusively to cytomorphology. *Essentials in Cytopathology* does not presume to replace any of the distinguished textbooks in cytopathology. Instead, the series will publish generously illustrated and user-friendly guides for both pathologists and clinicians.

Building on the amazing success of *The Bethesda System for Reporting Cervical Cytology*, now in its second edition, the *Series* will utilize a similar format, including minimal text, tabular criteria, and superb illustrations based on real-life specimens. *Essentials in Cytopathology* will, at times, deviate from the classic organization of pathology texts. The logic of decision trees, elimination of unlikely choices, and narrowing of differential diagnosis via a pragmatic approach based on morphologic criteria will be some of the strategies used to illustrate principles and practice in cytopathology.

Most of the authors for *Essentials in Cytopathology* are faculty members in The Johns Hopkins University School of Medicine, Department of Pathology, Division of Cytopathology. They bring to each volume the legacy of John K. Frost and the collective experience of a preeminent cytopathology service. The archives at Hopkins are meticulously catalogued and form the framework for text and illustrations. Authors from other institutions have been selected on the basis of their national reputations, experience, and enthusiasm for cytopathology. They bring to the series complementary viewpoints and enlarge the scope of materials contained in the photographs.

The editor and authors are indebted to our students, past and future, who challenge and motivate us to become the best that we possibly can be. We share that experience with you through these pages, and hope that you will learn from them as we have from those who have come before us. We would be remiss if we did not pay tribute to our professional colleagues, the cytotechnologists and preparatory technicians who lovingly care for the specimens that our clinical colleagues send to us.

And finally, we cannot emphasize enough throughout these volumes the importance of collaboration with the patient-care team. Every specimen comes to us as a question begging an answer. Without input from the clinicians, complete patient history, results of imaging studies, and other ancillary tests, we cannot perform optimally. It is our responsibility to educate our clinicians about their role in our interpretation, and for us to integrate as much information as we can gather into our final diagnosis, even if the answer at first seems obvious.

We hope you will find this series useful and welcome your feedback as you place these handbooks by your microscopes, and into your book bags.

Dorothy L. Rosenthal
Baltimore MD, USA
drosenthal@jhmi.edu

Contents

1
Introduction to Soft Tissue and Bone Cytopathology: A Practical Approach

Fine-needle aspiration cytology (FNAC) is increasingly becoming a widely accepted diagnostic modality for initial diagnoses, as well as, for recurrences and metastases of soft tissue lesions. Soft tissue lesions pose a challenge to diagnostic interpretation by FNAC.

FNAC in soft tissue lesions, as compared to open biopsy, is a simple, inexpensive outpatient procedure which is well tolerated by patients and has a minimal risk of complications (Table 1.1). Patient anxiety can be relieved by providing an instant diagnosis followed by discussion of management options. With thin needles it is easy to sample material from different parts of large tumors, thereby revealing possible tumor heterogeneity. To overcome the FNA limitation that tumor tissue architecture is better evaluated in surgical biopsies, we can evaluate these architectures to lesser degree in cell blocks prepared from specimens obtained by FNA. Cell block also provides an excellent material for additional ancillary studies if needed. Through rapid staining such as Diff Quick stain applied to aspiration smears it is possible to assess FNA specimen adequacy while the patient waits. If necessary, additional aspirations can be performed in order to obtain material for additional ancillary studies such as microbiological study, immunostain study, cytogenetic/fluorescence in-situ hybridization (FISH) study, and electron microscopy (EM) study.[2-10] However,

W.E. Khalbuss and A.V. Parwani, *Cytopathology of Soft Tissue and Bone Lesions*, Essentials in Cytopathology 9,
DOI 10.1007/978-1-4419-6499-1_1,
© Springer Science+Business Media, LLC 2011

TABLE 1.1.   Cost comparison FNA for palpable lesions vs. image-guidance vs. open biopsy.[1]

FNA of palpable lesions	$200
Image-guided FNA	$1,000
Open biopsy	$6,200

one disadvantage of FNAC is the occasional difficulty in obtaining sufficient material for ancillary studies, due to the nature of the lesion such as marked desmoplasia or fibrosis.

General FNA categories in Soft Tissue FNA (Geisinger & Abdul-Karim with Modifications)

Spindle Cell Lesions (Chapter 3)
* Fibromatosis
* Nodular fasciitis
* Spindle cell lipoma
* Schwannoma
* Neurofibroma
* Fibrosarcoma
* Synovial sarcoma
* Leiomyosarcoma
* MPNST
* Kaposi sarcoma
* Some MFH
* Some Angiosarcoma
* DFP

Myxoid Lesions (Chapter 5)
* Ganglion cyst
* Myxoma
* Nodular fasciitis
* Myxoid liposarcoma
* Myxoid MFH
* Myxoid chondrosarcoma
* Chordoma
* Metastatic mucinous Ca

Round Cell Lesions (Chapter 6)
* Paraganglioma
* Glomus tumor
* Solitary fibrous tumor
* Rhabdomyosarcoma
* Ewing/PNET
* Neuroblastoma
* DSRCT
* PD. synovial sarcoma
* Cellular variant of EMC
* Non-Hodgkin lymphoma

Polygonal/Epithelioid Lesions (Chapter 6)
* Rhabdomyoma
* Granular cell tumor
* Epithelioid sarcoma
* Epithelioid variants of leiomyosarcoma
* MPNST, epithelioid variant
* Angiosarcoma
* Epithelioid hemangioendothelioma
* Malignant extrarenal rhabdoid tumor
* Pleomorphic rhabdomyosarcoma
* Clear cell sarcoma
* Alveolar soft part sarcoma
* Metastatic tumors
* Some types of lymphomas

* DFP: Dermatofibrosarcoma protuberans
* EMC: Extraskeletal Myxoid Chondrosarcoma
* MFH: malignant fibrohistiocytoma
* MPNST: malignant peripheral nerve sheath tumor
* DSRCT: desmoplastic small round cell tumor.
* PNET: Primitive neuroectodermal tumor

FIG. 1.1.   General categories in soft tissue and bone FNA (From Geisinger and Abdul-Karim[11] with modifications).

Soft tissue gives rise to a wide variety of lesions having overlapping morphological appearance but with different biologic behavior. The integration of clinical and radiological findings with cytological findings cannot be overemphasized in reaching an accurate diagnosis. A practical cytomorphological approach for interpretation of FNAC of soft tissue lesions is to categorize the lesions based on the background of the smears and the predominance of cell type in the specimen[11] (Fig. 1.1). The background of the smears can be categorized into clean, inflammatory, myxoid/mucinous, collagenous/fibrotic, cartilaginous, osseous, hemorrhagic, and necrotic background (See Fig. 1.2). The predominant cell type can be categorized into: spindle cell, large round/polygonal cells, pleomorphic cells, small cells, inflammatory-type cells, and giant-cell containing (Fig. 1.3). Each of those categories presents certain differential diagnoses (Fig. 1.1). For example, smears with predominant small cell are easily recognized as neoplastic and malignant ancillary studies are required

---

General FNA categories in Soft Tissue FNA (Geisinger & Abdul-Karim with Modifications) (Continued from page 1)

Inflammatory/Reactive Cells (Chapter 6)
- Abscess
- Granulomatous inflammation
- Proliferative fasciitis/myositis
- Focal myositis
- Fat necrosis
- Muscle regeneration

Lipomatous Tumors (Chapter 7)
- Lipoma
- Fibrolipoma
- Chondroid lipoma
- Intramuscular lipoma
- Myelolipoma
- Hibernoma
- Liposarcoma
- Lipoblastoma

Pleomorphic Tumors (Chapters 4-7)
- MFH
- Pleomorphic sarcomas
  - Liposarcoma
  - Rhabdomyosarcoma
  - Other sarcomas

- MFH: malignant fibrohistiocytoma

Giant Cell Lesions (Chapter 4)
- Giant Cell Tumor of Tendon Sheath
- Myositis ossificans
- Giant Cell Tumor of Bone
- Fibrosarcoma/MFH
- Pleomorphic sarcoma:
- Giant Cell-Rich Osteosarcoma
- Metastatic pleomorphic carcinoma

FIG. 1.1. (continued)

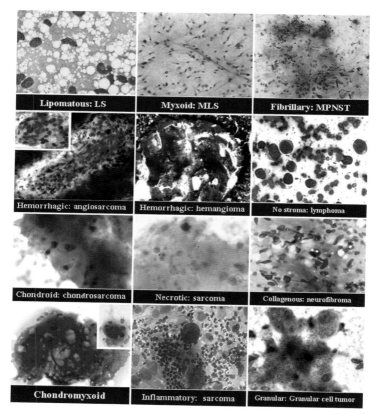

FIG. 1.2. Examples of categorization of background findings in soft tissue and bone FNAC. *LS* liposarcoma, *MLS* myxoid liposarcoma, and *MPNST* malignant peripheral nerve sheath tumor.

to establish a specific diagnosis. The morphologic evaluation can also be supplemented by ancillary techniques such as FISH, and immunocytochemistry. With integration of the clinical presentation, radiological findings, cytomorphological features, and ancillary studies (multidisciplinary approach), a specific diagnosis can be rendered in the majority of soft tissue lesions, with accuracy greater than 90% in most publications. However, in a

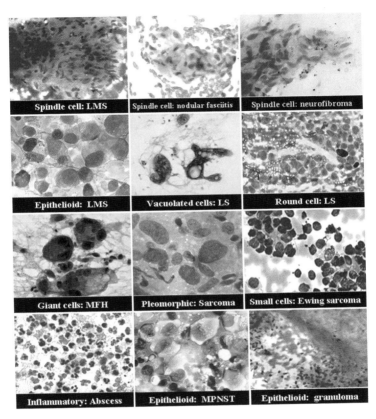

Fig. 1.3. Categorization of predominant cell type in soft tissue and bone FNAC. *LMS* leiomyosarcoma, *LS* liposarcoma, *MFH* malignant fibrous histiocytoma, and *MPNST* malignant peripheral nerve sheath tumor.

minority of cases, an inconclusive diagnosis (uncertain whether benign or malignant) may be encountered, in which the patient should be referred for tissue biopsy.

References

1. Layfield LJ. *Cytopathology of Bone and Soft Tissue Tumors.* New York: Oxford University Press; 2002:3–21.

2. Nagira K, Yamamoto T, Akisue T, et al. Reliability of fine-needle aspiration biopsy in the initial diagnosis of soft-tissue lesions. *Diagn Cytopathol*. 2002;27(6):354–361.

3. Khalbuss WE, Teot LA, Monaco SE. Diagnostic accuracy and limitations of fine needle aspiration cytology of bone and soft tissue lesions: a review of 1114 cases with cytological-histological correlation. *Cancer Cytopathol*. 2009;118(1):24–32.

4. Jorda M, Rey L, Hanly A, Ganjei-Azar P. Fine-needle aspiration cytology of bone: accuracy and pitfalls of cytodiagnosis. *Cancer*. 2000; 90(1):47–54.

5. Rekhi B, Gorad BD, Kakade AC, Chinoy R. Scope of FNAC in the diagnosis of soft tissue tumors – a study from a tertiary cancer referral center in India. *Cytojournal*. 2007;4:20.

6. García-Solano J, García-Rojo B, Sánchez-Sanchez C, Montalbán-Romero S, Martínez-Parra D, Pérez-Guillermo M. On the utility and limitations of fine-needle aspiration of palpable lesions located in the hand. *Diagn Cytopathol*. 2000;23(4):284–291.

7. Wakely PE Jr, Kneisl JS. Soft tissue aspiration cytopathology. *Cancer*. 2000;90(5):292–298.

8. Hirachand S, Lakhey M, Singha AK, Devkota S, Akhter J. Fine needle aspiration (FNA) of soft tissue tumors (STT). *Kathmandu Univ Med J (KUMJ)*. 2007;5(3):374–377.

9. Fleshman R, Mayerson J, Wakely PE Jr. Fine-needle aspiration biopsy of high-grade sarcoma: a report of 107 cases. *Cancer*. 2007;111(6): 491–498.

10. Handa U, Bal A, Mohan H, Bhardwaj S. Fine needle aspiration cytology in the diagnosis of bone lesions. *Cytopathology*. 2005;16(2): 59–64.

11. Geisinger KR, Abdul-Karim FW. Fine needle aspiration biopsies of soft tissue tumors. In: Weiss SW, Goldblum JR, eds. *Soft Tissue Tumors*. 4th ed. St Louise: C.V. Mosby Co; 2001:147–188.

2
Diagnostic Accuracy of FNA of Soft Tissue and Bone Lesions

The diagnosis of bone and soft tissue lesions can be obtained in a variety of ways, including FNA biopsy, core biopsy, or open biopsy. Each of these diagnostic tools has advantages and disadvantages. When compared to open biopsy, FNA is a simple, outpatient procedure which is well tolerated by patients and has minimal risk of complications. In addition, the multiple trajectories of the FNA biopsy needle make it possible to sample different parts of large tumors, opposed to a single small core biopsy or open biopsy. However, FNA biopsies can have sampling errors attributed to low cellularity, inadequate sampling of the target, and copious cystic/bloody/necrotic material.[1–3] Despite these difficulties, FNA cytology is being used as a diagnostic modality for initial diagnoses, as well as for recurrences and metastases of soft tissue and bone lesions in numerous medical centers due to its simplicity, low morbidity, cost-effectiveness, and ability to issue rapid diagnoses that can facilitate clinical decision making.[1–23]

There have been a large number of studies looking at the success and limitations of FNA biopsy in the setting of soft tissue and bone lesions. In at least 12 studies in the literature, the sensitivity has been reported to range from 25 to 100% and the specificity has ranged from 83 to 100% (Table 2.1).[1,2,4–13] Furthermore, many studies have had variable inadequacy rates that range from a low of 0–5% [2,3,14,22] to a high of 31–33% [4,23] raising concerns

W.E. Khalbuss and A.V. Parwani, *Cytopathology of Soft Tissue and Bone Lesions*, Essentials in Cytopathology 9, DOI 10.1007/978-1-4419-6499-1_2, © Springer Science+Business Media, LLC 2011

TABLE 2.1. Sensitivity and specificity of soft tissue and bone FNA in 12 studies.

Studies	Sensitivity (%)	Specificity (%)	Number of cases
Layfield et al[12]	95	95	N.A.
Bommer et al[11]	96	99	450
Wakely et al[10]	100	97	82
Garcia-Solano et al[9]	91	100	107
Jorda et al[4]	92	99	314
Nagira et al[1]	92	97	N.A.
Kitagawa et al[6]	100	100	93
Amin et al[5]	81	100	N.A.
Dey et al[8]	92	93	N.A.
Rekhi et al[7]	100	83	127
Hirachand et al[13]	25	100	50
Khalbuss et al[2]	97	98	1114

about the ability of FNA to obtain sufficient diagnostic material. The large variability in the reported sensitivities, specificities, and inadequacy rates is related to the variable number of cases available in the different studies, the type of lesions biopsied (soft tissue versus bone), the presence or absence of onsite evaluation, and other factors. Due to variability in the reported success of FNA, the use of this diagnostic tool in bone and soft tissue lesions has been fraught with some controversy, particularly in the setting of initial diagnoses of mesenchymal tumors.

Our data show a high overall sensitivity of 96% and specificity of 98% for the FNA diagnosis of soft tissue and bone lesions, and a very low rate (3%) of inadequacy, in the largest series of bone and soft tissue FNAs reported in the literature. The success of FNA in our practice may be attributable to the presence of a cytopathologist for onsite evaluation in the majority of cases and the presence of concurrent core biopsy in selected cases, which allows for optimization of the FNA in obtaining sufficient material and provides immediate cytological–histological correlation, respectively. In addition, our large volume of cases, including cases with a history of previous malignancy and/or supporting ancillary studies, has generated experience and familiarity with these challenging cases. A combination of all of these factors likely contributes to the high diagnostic sensitivity and specificity, in addition to minimizing our number of inadequate cases.

References

1. Nagira K, Yamamoto T, Akisue T, et al. Reliability of fine-needle aspiration biopsy in the initial diagnosis of soft-tissue lesions. *Diagn Cytopathol.* 2002;27(6):354–361.

2. Khalbuss WE, Teot LA, Monaco SE. Diagnostic accuracy and limitations of fine needle aspiration cytology of bone and soft tissue lesions: a review of 1114 cases with cytological-histological correlation. *Cancer Cytopathol.* 2009;118(1):24–32.

3. Akerman M, Rydholm A, Persson BM. Aspiration cytology of soft-tissue tumors. The 10-year experience at an orthopedic oncology center. *Acta Orthop Scand.* 1985;56:407–412.

4. Jorda M, Rey L, Hanly A, Ganjei-Azar P. Fine-needle aspiration cytology of bone: accuracy and pitfalls of cytodiagnosis. *Cancer.* 2000;90(1): 47–54.

5. Amin MS, Luqman M, Jamal S, Mamoon N, Anwar M. Fine needle aspiration biopsy of soft tissue tumors. *J Coll Physicians Surg Pak.* 2003;13(11):625–628.

6. Kitagawa Y, Ito H, Sawaizumi T, Matsubara M, Yokoyama M, Naito Z. Fine needle aspiration cytology for soft tissue tumours of the hand. *J Hand Surg Br.* 2003;28(6):582–585.

7. Rekhi B, Gorad BD, Kakade AC, Chinoy R. Scope of FNAC in the diagnosis of soft tissue tumors – a study from a tertiary cancer referral center in India. *Cytojournal.* 2007;4:20.

8. Dey P, Mallik MK, Gupta SK, Vasishta RK. Role of fine needle aspiration cytology in the diagnosis of soft tissue tumors and tumor like lesions. *Cytopathology.* 2004;15:32–37.

9. García-Solano J, García-Rojo B, Sánchez-Sánchez C, Montalbán-Romero S, Martínez-Parra D, Pérez-Guillermo M. On the utility and limitations of fine-needle aspiration of palpable lesions located in the hand. *Diagn Cytopathol.* 2000;23(4):284–291.

10. Wakely PE Jr, Kneisl JS. Soft tissue aspiration cytopathology. *Cancer.* 2000;90(5):292–298.

11. Bommer KK, Ramzy I, Mody D. Fine-needle aspiration biopsy in the diagnosis and management of bone lesions: a study of 450 cases. *Cancer.* 1997;81(3):148–56.

12. Layfield LJ, Anders KH, Glasgow BJ, Mira JM. Fine needle aspiration of primary soft-tissue tumors. *Arch Pathol Lab Med.* 1986;110:420–424.

13. Hirachand S, Lakhey M, Singha AK, Devkota S, Akhter J. Fine needle aspiration (FNA) of soft tissue tumours (STT). *Kathmandu Univ Med J (KUMJ).* 2007;5(3):374–377.

14. Kilpatrick SE, Cappellari JO, Bos GD, Gold SH, Ward WG. Is fine-needle aspiration biopsy a practical alternative to open biopsy for the primary diagnosis of sarcoma? *Am J Clin Pathol.* 2001;115:59–68.

15. Maitra A, Ashfaq R, Hossein Saboorian M, Lindberg G, Gokasian S. The role of fine-needle aspiration biopsy in the primary diagnosis of mesenchymal lesions. A community hospital-based experience. *Cancer*. 2000;3:178–185.

16. Domanski HA, Gustafson P. Cytologic features of primary, recurrent, and metastatic dermatofibrosarcoma protuberans. *Cancer*. 2002;96: 351–361.

17. Layfield LJ. Cytologic diagnosis of osseous lesions: a review with emphasis on the diagnosis of primary neoplasms of bone. *Diagn Cytopathol*. 2009;37(4):299–310.

18. Fleshman R, Mayerson J, Wakely PE Jr. Fine-needle aspiration biopsy of high-grade sarcoma: a report of 107 cases. *Cancer*. 2007;111(6): 491–498.

19. Sápi Z, Antal I, Pápai Z, et al. Diagnosis of soft tissue tumors by fine-needle aspiration with combined cytopathology and ancillary techniques. *Diagn Cytopathol*. 2002;26(4):232–242.

20. Handa U, Bal A, Mohan H, Bhardwaj S. Fine needle aspiration cytology in the diagnosis of bone lesions. *Cytopathology*. 2005;16(2):59–64.

21. Domanski HA, Akerman M, Carlén B, et al. Core-needle biopsy performed by the cytopathologist: a technique to complement fine-needle aspiration of soft tissue and bone lesions. *Cancer*. 2005;105(4): 229–239.

22. Layfield LJ, Glasgow BJ, Anders KH, Mirra JM. Fine needle aspiration cytology of primary bone lesions. *Acta Cytol*. 1987;31(2):177–184.

23. Dollahite HA, Tatum L, Moinuddin SM, Carnesale PG. Aspiration biopsy of primary neoplasms of bone. *J Bone Joint Surg*. 1989;71: 1166–1169.

3
Cytopathology of Spindle Cell Lesions of Soft Tissue and Bone

Spindle cell lesions of soft tissue and bone encompass a wide spectrum of benign and malignant conditions. They include reactive lesions such as granulomatous inflammation, pseudosarcomas such as nodular fasciitis, benign mesenchymal tumors such as neurofibroma and schwannoma, low and high-grade sarcomas, spindle cell carcinoma, and spindle cell melanoma. The sarcomas that can be presented as spindle cells include fibrosarcoma (FS), leiomyosarcoma (LMS), synovial sarcoma, malignant peripheral nerve sheath tumor (MPNST), Kaposi sarcoma, low-grade fibromyxoid sarcoma, gastrointestinal stromal tumor (GIST), and some angiosarcomas[1,2] (Table 3.1).

The wide spectrum of spindle cell lesions of soft tissue and bone presents diagnostic challenges to cytologists due to overlapping morphologic appearances of reactive and neoplastic lesions and makes it susceptible to misdiagnosis. The phenomenon of pseudotumors has long been recognized in histopathology with commentary on adverse consequences for over interpretation. Low-grade sarcomas may have relatively bland cytological features, hence separation of these sarcomas from pseudosarcomas can be extremely challenging. Illustrations of such entities will be seen throughout this chapter.

W.E. Khalbuss and A.V. Parwani, *Cytopathology of Soft Tissue and Bone Lesions*, Essentials in Cytopathology 9,
DOI 10.1007/978-1-4419-6499-1_3,
© Springer Science+Business Media, LLC 2011

TABLE 3.1. The differential diagnosis of soft tissue and bone tumors with spindle cell morphology.

Benign	Malignant
Nodular fasciitis/pseudosarcoma	Fibrosarcoma
Schwannoma/neurofibroma	Leiomyosarcoma
Spindle cell lipoma/fibrolipoma	Synovial sarcoma
Leiomyoma	Malignant peripheral nerve sheath tumors (MPNST)
Fibromatosis	Kaposi sarcoma
Granulomatous inflammation	Low-grade fibromyxoid sarcoma
	Gastrointestinal stromal tumor (GIST)
	Some angiosarcomas
	Some liposarcomas
	Malignant Fibrous Histiocytoma (MFH)
	Metastatic spindle cell carcinoma
	Malignant spindle cell melanoma

Granulomatous Inflammation with Spindle Cell Morphology[3,4] (Fig. 3.1)

Cytomorphology

- Aggregates of epithelioid histiocytes with elongated "Sandal-like" nuclei without nuclear polarity.
- Scanty inflammatory cells and multinucleated giant cells.
- Necrotic debris and caseation if the granuloma is necrotizing.

Differential Diagnosis

- Infectious etiology: mycobacterial, fungal and others.

Ancillary Studies

- CD68+, CK(−), AFB, GMS.
- Non-infectious etiology: e.g., sarcoidosis.
- Malignancies associated: nodular sclerosis of Hodgkin lymphoma and seminoma.

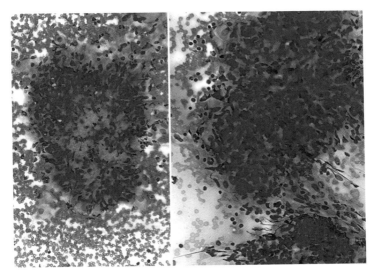

Fᴵɢ. 3.1. Granulomatous inflammation of soft tissue. Multiple aggregates of epithelioid histiocytes with elongated "Sandal-like" nuclei without nuclear polarity, few lymphocytes, and multinucleated giant cells. (DQ stain, left x100, right x200). The GMS and AFB stains on cell block were negative. Microbiological cultures from FNA material were negative. The findings were suggestive of sarcoidosis.

Pseudosarcomas (Nodular Fasciitis, Myositis Ossificans, and Proliferative Fasciitis[5]) (Figs. 3.2 and 3.3)

- Relatively common soft tissue tumors, often mistaken for sarcomas.
- A rapidly enlarging mass in adults, third to fourth decade.
- Mimics sarcoma, synonymous with pseudosarcomatous and infiltrative fasciitis.
- Occasionally is associated with trauma in 10–15%.
- The most common location is the forearm, but can be in a variety of locations.
- Subtypes: subcutaneous (most common), intramuscular, and fascial.
- May regress spontaneously.

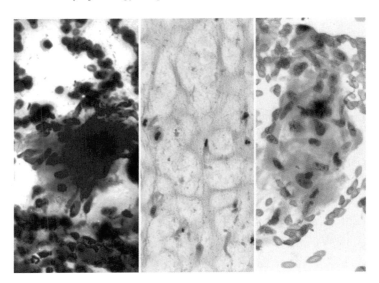

FIG. 3.2. Nodular fasciitis presented as rapidly growing shoulder mass (*left DQ stain*, 400, *middle and right Pap stain*, ×200 and ×400). There are mixed patterns in the same lesion that include myxoid and non-myxoid, hypocellular and hypercellular areas of bland-appearing spindle cells and some scattered lymphocytes. Excisional biopsy: nodular fasciitis.

Histological Features

- The typical histologic features include tissue culture-like fibroblasts with abundant mitoses, arranged in short bundles within a variably myxoid matrix.
- Frequently considered to be a pseudosarcoma due to its rapid growth and high mitotic activity which makes it difficult to distinguish from a spindle cell sarcoma.

Cytomorphology of Pseudosarcomas

- Mixed cytomorphological patterns (myxoid, edematous, bone tissue, inflammatory cells, hypocellular areas, and hypercellular areas).

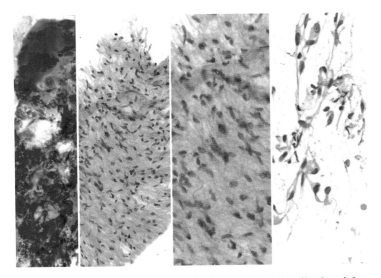

FIG. 3.3. Myositis ossificans with predominance of spindle cells (*from left to right*: DQ smears, ×200, Pap stained smears ×200, ×400, ×400, respectively). The smears show predominance of bland-appearing spindle cells with smooth nuclear membranes and evenly distributed chromatin and granular and fibrillar background. Also seen are numerous plasmacytoid cells (*right*) and bone tissue with osteoblasts and multinucleated osteoclasts (*left*). The excisional biopsy confirmed the diagnosis of myositis ossificans with zonations of the lesion including peripheral zone, the bony trabeculae.

- The proliferating cells are a mixture (spindle, stellate fibroblasts, polygonal mimic ganglion cells, and inflammatory cells). However, they are mainly spindle with dense fields and with cellular overlapping (Figs. 3.2 and 3.3).
- The spindle shapes have a small to moderate amount of pale staining cytoplasm.
- Nuclei in relatively uniform sizes and shape, oval/elongated/finely granular chromatin, and smooth or curved nuclear contours.
- Nucleoli are generally inconspicuous; occasionally, small nucleoli can be seen.
- Inflammatory cells (lymphocytes), extravasated red blood cells, occasional giant cells, and a minor population of cells with polygonal, stellate features.

- Metachromatic-staining myxoid material and occasional granular background.
- No or rare mitotic figures, no necrotic debris, and no intranuclear inclusions.
- Long-standing lesions can have more of a fibrotic or hyalinized appearance, whereas the lesions with a more myxoid appearance are usually new or recent lesions. Therefore, older lesions may be more difficult to aspirate.
- Proliferative fasciitis is characterized by large ganglion-like cells.
- Proliferative myositis often exhibits multinucleated regenerating muscle fibers.
- Myositis ossificans (Fig. 3.3) may contain bone tissue.

Differential Diagnosis

- Benign and malignant neoplastic lesions (one population of cells with monomorphic pattern), Desmoid type fibromatosis (cell population is less pleomorphic).

Ancillary Studies

- Vimentin +, MSA (+), calponin (+)
- Cytokeratin (−), S100 (−), and CD34 (−), desmin (−), caldesmon (−).

Summary and Key Features

- Rapidly growing spindle cell lesion in adults showing mixed cytomorphological patterns (spindle, stellate fibroblast, polygonal, inflammatory; myxoid, edematous, dense, hypo and hypercellular, and/or bone tissue).

Benign Neurgogenic Tumor[6,7] (Schwannoma and Neurofibroma) (Fig. 3.4)

- Schwannoma is a benign tumor of peripheral nerves composed exclusively of Schwann cells with nerve at the periphery of the tumor.

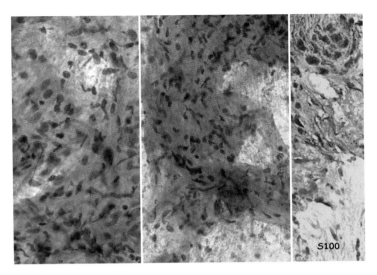

FIG. 3.4. FNA of neurogenic tumor from 21-year-old female who presented with 2 cm soft tissue mass in the deltoid area. Smears (Pap stain ×400 and S100 immunostain ×200, *right*) showed spindle-cell proliferative lesion with elongated wavy irregular nuclei with pointed ends. The chromatin is bland and the nucleoli are not prominent. Immunostain on cell block material shows positivity for S100 (diffuse and strong). The cytological diagnosis was neurogenic tumor, neurofibroma vs. schwannoma. The follow-up surgical excision was schwannoma.

- Schwannoma is most common in adults as a subcutaneous, less often intramuscular tumor.
- Neurofibroma is composed of all nerve components: Schwann cells, nerve axons, fibroblasts and perineural cells with nerve often penetrating the center of NF. Tumor presents anywhere in the body.
- It can be superficial, protrude from skin or be a deeper tumor.
- Malignant change in neurofibroma occurs in about 10% of deep-seated tumors of extremities or neck, almost always in fibromatosis I.

Cytomorphology of Neurofibroma/Schwannoma

- Aspiration is often painful and can yield non-diagnostic material when the needle hits collagenized areas, myxoid, or cystic degeneration.
- Aspirates show numerous bland, spindly, comma, and bullet-shaped cells inside the large irregular tissue fragments. Sometimes Verocay bodies are seen.
- Ancient schwannomas may show a focal marked nuclear pleomorphism with uncommon mitotic figures.
- Variable cellularity with most cells forming cohesive clusters, few are dispersed.
- Cells are spindle shaped with elongated nuclei and exhibit characteristics of wavy irregular nuclei with pointed ends and fibroblasts.
- Chromatin is bland and nucleoli are not prominent.
- The background is frequently myxoid.
- Contrary to MPNST, schwannoma/neurofibroma shows diffuse and strong positivity with S-100.

Ancillary Studies

- Vimentin+, S100 + (diffuse and strong), SMA−, Desmin−.

Differential Diagnosis

- Nodular fasciitis (mixed cytomorphological patterns);
- MPNST (atypia with coarse and hyperchromatic chromatin and focally positive for S-100);
- LMS (nuclei are plumper, desmin+, smooth muscle actin+).

Spindle Cell Lipoma[8,9] (Fig. 3.5)

- Well-circumscribed subcutaneous lesions on the neck, back, and shoulder.
- More common in older males.

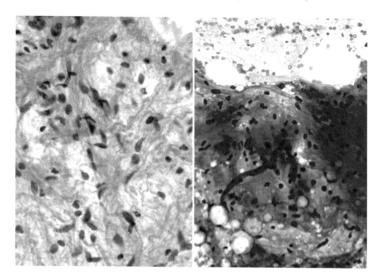

FIG. 3.5. Fibrolipoma: the lesion was a well-circumscribed subcutaneous neck tumor. It shows mixture of mature adipose tissue and bland spindle cells in a myxoid and collagenous background. (*Left*, Pap stain, x200, *right* DQ stain x100). FISH study was done on this case and it was negative for genetic changes of a myxoid liposarcoma.

- Cytomorphology of Spindle Cell Lipoma Aspirates of spindle cell lipomas usually present as a mixture of mature adipose tissue associated with dispersed or clustered bland spindle cells.
- Myxoid background is common with eosinophilic collagen – hyaline fibers and mast cells.
- Pleomorphic lipoma shows variable number of bizarre pleomorphic giant cells with dark nuclei, on occasion forming rings ("floret cells").

Differential Diagnosis

- Myxoid sarcoma: Myxoid liposarcoma (deep-seated and branching capillaries and lipoblasts) Low-grade myxofibrosarcoma (deep-seated and coarse vessel fragments).

- Ancillary Studies Schwannoma: spindle cells (S-100+ and CD34−).
- Atypical lipomatous tumor/well-differentiated liposarcoma (deep-seated and occasional lipoblasts).

Solitary Fibrous Tumor [4,10] (Fig. 3.6)

- An uncommon tumor affecting adults and occasionally children.
- It is located superficially and in deep soft tissues of various locations: extremities, head and neck, thoracic wall, retroperitoneum, mediastinum.
- Most cases are benign, some are malignant.
- In histological sections there are hypocellular and hypercellular areas of small round and spindle cells, bands of hyalinized stroma, and branching vascular spaces (hemangiopericytoma pattern).

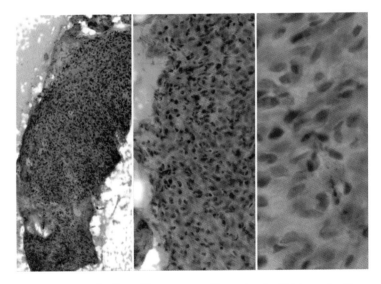

FIG. 3.6. FNA of solitary fibrous tumor. The patient had history of solitary fibrous tumor of leg and presented with a mass in the same location. The smears (Pap stains ×100, ×200, and ×400) show one population of spindle cells and round cells presented as larger tissue fragments. The immunostain on cell block material shows vimentin and CD34 positivity confirming recurrence of solitary fibrous tumor.

- In malignant tumors there is high cellularity, numerous mitoses, necrosis, and atypia.

Cytomorphology of Solitary Fibrous Tumor

- Predominance of spindle cells or a mixture of spindle and round cells.
- Cell groups, dissociated cells, and naked nuclei are present in variable numbers.
- When larger tissue fragments are present they contain numerous capillaries.
- Tumor cells are round, medium sized with scant cytoplasm.
- Some cells appear plasmacytoid due to peripheral location of nuclei.
- It is not possible to differentiate benign solitary fibrous tumors from malignant ones because malignant tumors often lack atypia.

Ancillary Studies

Imunohistochemistry: CD34+, CD99+, EMA+/−, BCL2+/−, SMA+/−, and S100+/−.

Aneurysmal Bone Cyst[11–13] (Fig. 3.7)

- Uncommon lesion.
- Radiology is characteristic: ballooning of the bone contour (soap bubble appearance).
- Young age: 1–20 years (80%) with recurrence in 20%.
- May be secondary to trauma or arise in preexisting bone lesion (giant cell tumor, chondroblastoma, fibrous dysplasia).
- Benign lesion; grows rapidly, multiloculated locally aggressive cystic neoplasm. Rarely transforms to osteosarcoma.
- Expanding osteolytic lesion of blood-filled spaces of variable size separated by connective tissue septa with osteoclast giant cells and variable reactive bone.

Cytomorphology of Aneurysmal Bone Cyst

- Cysts and septa lined by fibroblasts, myofibroblasts, and histiocytes but not endothelium.

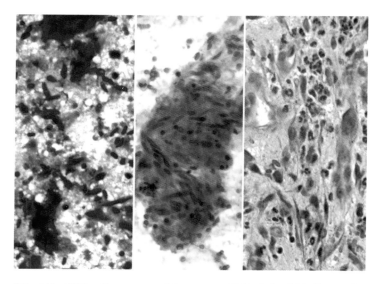

FIG. 3.7. FNA of aneurysmal bone cyst (DQ, *left* ×200; Pap stain, *middle*, ×200, and cell block, *right* H&E ×400): Clusters of osteoclast-like multinucleated giant cells with loose spindly stroma to cellular stroma. The cell block, *right* shows fragments of bland-appearing fibroconnective tissue with fibroblasts, myofibroblasts, histiocytes, and giant cells but not endothelium; no malignant osteoid, no atypia. The excisional biopsy of this lesion showed aneurysmal bone cyst with infarction.

- Clusters of osteoclast-like multinucleated giant cells with loose spindly stroma to cellular stroma.
- Reactive woven bone, degenerated calcifying fibromyxoid tissue; variable mitotic figures and hemosiderin; no malignant osteoid, no atypia. Ancillary Studies
- Molecular: abnormalities of 17p13.2 loci in 63%.

Differential Diagnosis

Solitary bone cyst, Giant cell tumor (lacks fibroblastic cells), Hemangioma, Telangiectatic osteosarcoma (more atypia), Giant cell reparative granuloma (if in jaw), Low-grade osteosarcoma (hypocellular).

Leiomyosarcoma[14–16] (Fig. 3.8)

- Most seen as intra-abdominal lesions in the retroperitoneum, pelvis, mesentery, and omentum and account for 30–50% of sarcomas.
- Remaining LMS are divided into subcutaneous/deep soft tissue, cutaneous, and vascular groups.
- Subcutaneous or deep soft tissue LMS arise in limbs, especially in the thigh in middle-aged patients.
- Cutaneous LMS arise in younger adults in limbs, are often painful and frequently recur. Vascular LMS arise in older adults adjacent to blood vessels with muscular walls, in particular the inferior vena cava and the large veins of the lower extremity.

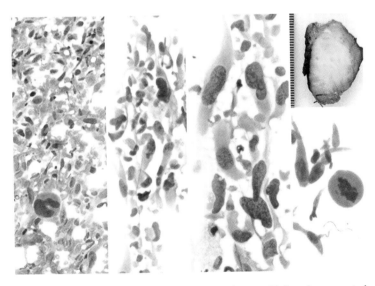

FIG. 3.8. FNA of leiomyosarcoma from 76-year-old female presented with deltoid mass (Pap stain, *from left to right* ×100, ×200, and ×400 and subsequent excisional biopsy, *right upper*). Atypical spindle cells with cigar-shaped nuclei and occasional perinuclear vacuoles. The nuclei show irregular coarse chromatin, pleomorphism, and increased mitotic activity.

Cytomorphology of Leiomyosarcoma

- Spindle cells may be deceptively bland.
- Nuclear atypia, mitotic activity, and irregular coarse chromatin.
- Fascicles of monomorphic spindle cells very often exhibit cigar-shaped nuclei with perinuclear vacuoles.
- Chromatin is finely granular, nucleoli are not prominent.
- Palisading of nuclei is common and single cells are rare.

Differential Diagnosis

- Leiomyoma (no atypia, no mitotic activity, and no necrosis); Pleomorphic liposarcoma (few lipoblasts and/or cytoplasmic vacuoles); Epithelioid sarcoma;
- Ancient schwannoma; and Rhabdomyosarcoma.

Myxofibrosarcoma/Myxoid MFH[17–19] (Fig. 3.9)

- One of the most common soft tissue sarcomas in adults.
- Subtypes: pleomorphic, myxoid, giant cell, and inflammatory.
- Myxoid MFH is the second most common variant, after the pleomorphic subtype.
- Usually in older adults in the extremities or retroperitoneum.
- Usually superficial with no gender predilection.
- Some lesions arise in the setting of orthopedic implants, Paget's disease, fibrous dysplasia, and bone infarcts.
- Associated with pathologic fracture in 25% of cases.
- Metaphyseal regions of long bones are the most frequently involved, as ill-defined lytic lesions with cortical expansion and breakthrough with minimal periosteal reaction.
- The superficial nature of this neoplasm can be a helpful distinguishing feature from the other myxoid soft tissue lesions that tend to be in deeper locations.
- Can metastasize to lymph nodes (same as synovial sarcoma, clear cell sarcoma, rhabdomyosarcoma).

Cytomorphology of Myxoid MFH

- The atypical cells can vary from bland-appearing in the low-grade lesions, to more pleomorphic in the high-grade lesions.

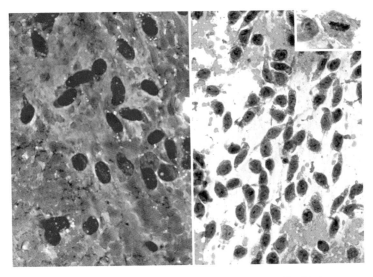

Fig. 3.9.   FNA of fibromyxoid sarcoma/myxoid malignant fibrohistiocytoma, MFH (DQ smear, *left* ×400, Pap stain smear, *right*, ×400) presented as sacral mass from a 79-year-old-male. The smears are abundantly cellular and demonstrate single and small loosely cohesive clusters of atypical spindle cells in an abundant myxoid background. The cells display pleomorphism. Nuclei have an irregular coarse chromatin distribution. Some cells showed vacuolated cytoplasm. Also seen are a high number of mitotic figures (insert, *right*).

- Abundant myxoid material may be present with vacuolated cells.
- The atypical cells may mimic lipoblasts or fibroblasts.
- Low-grade cases can mimic myxomas.
- Elongated fibroblast-like cells and histiocyte-like cells.

Differential Diagnosis

- Other sarcomas: FS,
- Liposarcomas,
- LMS,
- Chondrosarcoma.
- Benign fibrohistiocytic tumors: no malignant cells.

Summary/Key Features

- Superficial tumor in adults with elongated fibroblast-like cells and histiocyte-like cells and giant cells with nuclear atypia and possible myxoid background.

Fibrosarcoma[15,20] (Fig. 3.10)

- A rare malignant tumor composed of atypical fibroblasts.
- Variable collagen production and no other matrix production are allowed, resulting in a diagnosis of exclusion.
- Majority of the cases diagnosed in the past would be now classified as synovial sarcomas (which would stain with epithelial

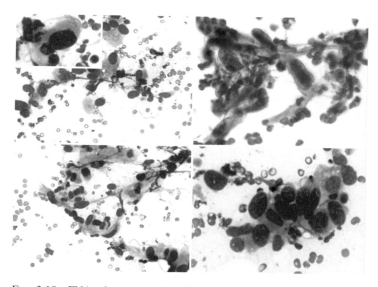

FIG. 3.10. FNA of post-radiation fibrosarcoma. The patient previously had radiation treatment for papillary carcinoma of the thyroid who developed neck mass. The specimen shows spindle-shaped pleomorphic cells arranged in small clusters and singly. The nuclei are fusiform, atypical with significant pleomorphism and with dark coarse chromatin. (*Left upper*, DQ stain x200, inset x 400; *right upper*, Pap stain x400; *lower left*, DQ x200; *lower right*, DQ x400).

markers and CD99), or MPNST (which would stain at least focally with S-100).

- It presents as a deep soft tissue mass in extremities, trunk, head, and neck in elderly patients.
- Prognosis is bad, with 10–60% of patients presenting with metastases of lung and bones. Five-year survival rate is about 50%.

Cytomorphology of Fibrosarcoma

- Atypical spindle-shaped cell population arranged in small clusters and singly.
- Nuclei are fusiform; atypia is variable, with dark coarse chromatin and prominent nucleoli in higher-grade lesions.
- Cytoplasm is elongated.

Differential Diagnosis

Monophasic fibrous synovial sarcoma (pan CK+ and EMA+); and MPNST (S100+).

Osteosarcoma[21–24] (Fig. 3.11)

- Soft tissue osteosarcomas account for <1% of all soft tissue sarcomas, and affect older patients (50–60s), in contrast to osseous osteosarcoma which occurs in young adults.
- Typically in proximal extremities as painless large mass.
- Most patient die of disease with up to 85% of patients developing metastasis.

Cytomorphology of Osteosarcoma

- Moderate to abundant cellularity with a background rich in red blood cells.
- Single and in clusters with marked nuclear atypia (hyperchromasia, irregular nuclear membrane and variation in cell size and shape, prominent nucleoli, and atypical mitoses).
- Osteosarcoma displays features of high-grade malignant pleomorphic sarcomas.
- Osteosarcoma is distinguished from other high-grade sarcomas by the presence of neoplastic bone and osteoid matrix formation in

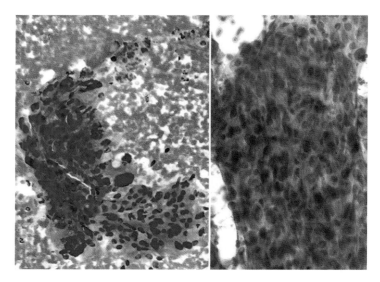

FIG. 3.11. FNA of osteosarcoma (DQ stain, *left* ×300, and Pap stain, *right* ×400): the smears are cellular and show numerous clusters of large spindle cells (three to ten times the size of a red blood cell) displaying nuclear hyperchromasia, irregular nuclear membranes, and marked pleomorphism. Some neoplastic cells show plasmacytoid appearance with eccentric hyperchromatic nuclei, multinucleation, and occasional mitoses. The background is mostly hemorrhagic.

close association with the malignant osteoblasts in the absence of other lines of differentiation and appropriate radiographic setting.

- Osteoid is variably present, and best seen in Romanowsky-stained preparations where it can form aggregates or lace-like structures containing pleomorphic cells. Other features include presence of multinucleated neoplastic cells, and cells with eccentric nuclei akin to plasmacytoid appearance with variable presence of a paranuclear clear "hof."

Differential Diagnosis

- Pleomorphic sarcomas (MFH),
- Liposarcoma,
- Rhabdomyosarcoma,
- LMS.

Ancillary Studies

- Alkaline phosphatase, osteocalcin, and osteonectin are helpful in the diagnosis.

Angiosarcoma[25,26] (Fig. 3.12)

- Rare malignant vascular neoplasm that can arise in any part of the body.
- Most common location is in the skin of the head and neck region, soft tissues, and numerous solid organs.
- Divided into classical (spindle cell) and epithelioid subtypes.

Cytomorphology of Angiosarcoma

- Round, oval, spindle, and epithelioid cells.
- Single cells, pseudoacinar and rosette-like formations, papillary structures, and well-formed small vessels may be seen.

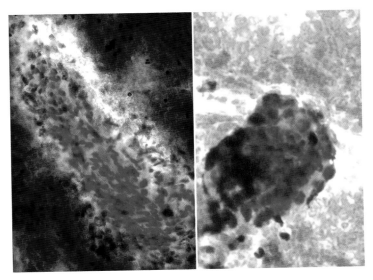

FIG. 3.12.   FNA of angiosarcoma (DQ stain ×300, *left*, and ×400, *right*): Highly atypical spindle cells with pleomorphic, eccentric, smooth and hyperchromatic nuclei, and prominent nucleoli. Cytoplasm is scanty and the background is hemorrhagic.

- Pleomorphism and hyperchromasia are often pronounced.
- Nucleoli can be conspicuous, large or multiple.
- Occasional nuclear folds, indentations, grooves, and mitotic figures.
- Cytoplasm is scant to moderate, may contain hemosiderin deposits, multiple small vacuoles or intracytoplasmic lumina.

Ancillary Studies

- Immunostain: CD31+, CD34+, and factor VIII+.

Differential Diagnosis

- Granulation tissue,
- Hemangioma,
- Kaposi's sarcoma;
- Dermatofibrosarcoma protuberans;
- MPNST,
- LMS,
- Low-grade myxofibrosarcoma,
- Monophasic synovial sarcoma, and
- Spindle cell liposarcoma.

Kaposi Sarcoma[22,27] (Fig. 3.13)

- First described in 1872, Kaposi sarcoma (KS) has four different epidemiological subgroups at high risk:
    - *Classic or European form* – elderly males with increased incidence in Ashkenazi Jews and persons of Mediterranean descent, usually involving the lower legs.
    - *African or endemic form* – children with typically fatal disease and young to middle-aged adults with benign nodular disease (originally had highest incidence in Zaire and Uganda).
    - *Iatrogenic form associated with immunosuppression* – aggressive disease in transplant patients which regresses with discontinuation of immunosuppression.
    - *AIDS-associated or epidemic form* – 300 times greater incidence of KS in AIDS patients compared to other immunosuppressed

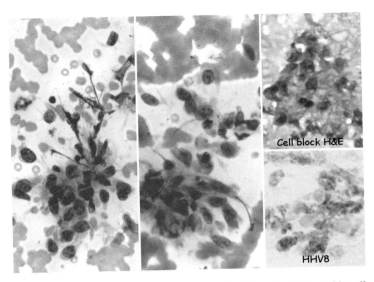

FIG. 3.13. FNA of kaposi sarcoma (DQ stain *left* and *middle*, ×400, cell block (H&E stain), ×400, and Human Herpes Virus type 8 immunostain, ×400, *right lower*). The patient was 36-year-old HIV-positive male patient who presented with brown irregular leg nodule. The smears demonstrate a bloody background with clusters of neoplastic spindle cells with ovoid nuclei with mostly smooth contours and finely-dispersed chromatin. Some nuclei display 1–2 small nucleoli and the characteristic nuclear streak artifact. Some neoplastic cells have a loose stroma and their cytoplasm forms tapered tails. There is mild nuclear pleomorphism. The spindle cells exhibit immunoreactivity with HHV8 (*right lower*).

patients before implementation of anti-retrovirals; lesions often over chest and face.
- Three recognized clinical disease patterns:
  – *Nodular* – circumscribed, cutaneous and subcutaneous nodules, indolent course though asymptomatic internal involvement is often present at death.
  – *Aggressive* – arises from background of pre-existing nodular disease which evolves into extensive exophytic and ulcerative or deep infiltrative growth usually involving the extremities (osseous and visceral involvement commonly present).

- *Generalized* – lymphadenopathic disease with or without systemic involvement primarily in children.
- AIDS-related KS may appear with any pattern, but usually in those with advanced immune suppression and CD4+T-cell counts <500 cells/mm^3.
- Though many agents have been implicated, human herpesvirus 8 (HHV 8) has been isolated from both HIV-associated and non-HIV-associated KS lesions.

Cytomorphology of Kaposi Sarcoma

- No well-defined morphologic differences between classical, endemic, iatrogenic, and AIDS-associated forms of KS.
- Smears have scanty cellularity with a bloody background. Scattered tissue fragments comprised of loosely cohesive clusters of spindle cells are seen. Resembling granulomas, the stroma is metachromatic on Romanowsky stain.
- The spindle cells are bland with large, oval nuclei with smooth contours, evenly dispersed chromatin, and usually inconspicuous nucleoli. The neoplastic cells have mild pleomorphism, indistinct cell borders, and prominent nuclear streak artifact.
- Cytoplasm is moderate and delicate and typically forms tapering tails which blend with that of the adjacent cells. Hyalines globules are occasionally present.

Ancillary Studies

Factor VIII+ related antigen, CD31+, CD34+, thrombomodulin+, and HHV-8+ (Kaposi sarcoma-associated herpes virus) in almost 100% of cases.

Differential Diagnosis

- Granulation tissue,
- Nodular fasciitis,
- Leiomyoma,
- Myofibroblastoma,
- Angiosarcoma,
- Spindle-cell malignant melanoma.

Malignant Peripheral Nerve Sheath Tumor[28,29] (Fig. 3.14)

- Also known as malignant schwannoma.
- Bulky deep-seated tumor usually arising from major nerves in neck, forearm, lower leg, and buttock.
- Fifty percent associated with neurofibromatosis (NF), 50% arise de novo.
- May be due to radiation; rarely arise from ganglioneuromas.
- Recur locally, distant metastases frequent.

Cytomorphology of MPNST

- Spindle cell neoplastic proliferation with a prominent collagenous component.

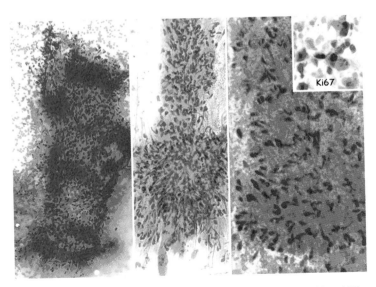

FIG. 3.14. FNA of MPNST (DQ stain ×100, *left*, Pap Stain ×200, *middle*, and Pap stain ×400, *right*). Smears show spindle cell proliferation with a prominent collagenous component. The spindle nuclei have tapered ends and a wavy appearance, suggestive of a neural origin; with immunostain for Ki67, >80% of tumor nuclei are immunoreactive.

- The tumor cells contained spindle nuclei with tapered ends and a wavy appearance, suggestive of a neural origin.
- The cells are monomorphic serpentine cells, with palisading.
- Necrosis and frequent mitotic figures may be seen.
- Fifteen percent may have metaplastic cartilage, bone, muscle.

Ancillary Studies

S100+, CD57+ , p53+, collagen IV+, CD99/O13+; EMA−, CK−; and t(X;18) negative

Differential Diagnosis

- Pleomorphic liposarcoma,
- MFH,
- Synovial sarcoma.

Spindle Cell Melanoma[30,31] (Fig. 3.15)

- Spindle cell melanoma (including desmoplastic melanoma) is a morphologic variant of melanoma.
- Incidence varies from 3 to 14%.
- May mimic other spindle cell lesions.
- May lack cytologic atypia.
- May show discrepancy in cell type between metastatic spindle cell melanomas and the primary epithelioid melanoma.

Cytomorphology of Spindle Cell Melanoma

- Highly cellular and contain mainly dissociated cells.
- Cell groups without organoid structure and accidental groupings are scarce or absent.
- Morphology of melanoma varies greatly from round, polygonal to spindle and some smears contain a mixture of all shapes.
- Melanoma with epithelioid or plasmacytoid morphology is rather common: abundant, well-demarcated cytoplasm, eccentric nuclei, and many binucleated and multinucleated cells. Melanin is usually absent or present only in occasional cells.

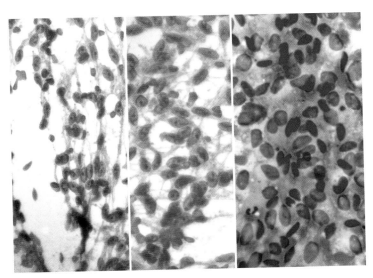

FIG. 3.15.   FNA of spindle cell melanoma (Pap stain, *left and middle* ×300 and ×400, DQ ×400, *right*). Patient with history of malignant melanoma presented with soft tissue neck mass. The cells are arranged singly and in clusters. The cell are spindle and epithelioid with some of plasmacytoid morphology. The cytoplasm is abundant and well demarcated. Some binucleation is noted. Melanin is seen in one cell as *dark blue/black* pigment (*right upper*).

Ancillary Studies

- HMB45+, Melan A+, and S-100+ (good marker except in separating melanoma from clear cell sarcoma).

Differential Diagnosis

- Malignant fibrohistiocytoma,
- FS,
- MPNST,
- LMS,
- Synovial sarcoma,
- Clear cell sarcoma,
- Pleomorphic carcinoma.

Pleomorphic/Spindle Cell Carcinoma[32,33] (Fig. 3.16)

- Pleomorphic/spindle cell carcinomas are high-grade carcinomas that are seen in many organs such as lung, pancreas, thyroid, and ovaries.
- May mimic other spindle cell lesions.
- Usually are pleomorphic, with necrosis and anaplastic features.

Cytomorphology of Spindle Cell Carcinoma

- Highly cellular and contain mainly dissociated cells.
- Single and clusters of markedly pleomorphic cells with spindle and giant cell features.
- Epithelioid, plasmacytoid, spindle cell, or giant cell/bizarre cell morphology.

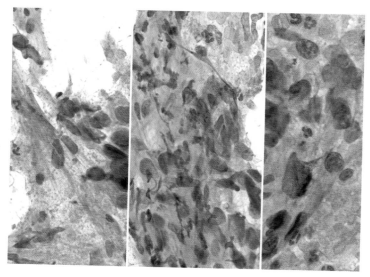

Fig. 3.16. Metastatic undifferentiated carcinoma of ovarian origin. The patient presented with soft tissue abdominal wall lesion. The smears (Pap stain, ×400) are highly cellular and contain dissociated spindle pleomorphic cells and cell groups without organoid structure associated with necrosis. The pan cytokeratin immunostain is positive confirming the epithelial origin of this neoplasm.

Ancillary Studies

- CK+

Differential Diagnosis

- Pleomorphic sarcomas,
- Spindle cell/pleomorphic melanoma.

Summary

See Table 3.2

TABLE 3.2. FNA of spindle cell lesions of soft tissue and bone.

Entity	Key cytological features
Pseudosarcoma, nodular fasciitis; myositis ossificans	No atypia, mixed cellular and background patterns
Schwannoma	Fishhook naked nuclei, spindle cells, Verocay bodies (palisading)
Neurofibroma	Fishhook naked nuclei, spindle cells, no Verocay bodies
Spindle cell lipoma/ fibrolipoma	Mixture of mature adipose tissue and bland spindle cells in a myxoid and collagenous background
Sarcomas	Mononuclear cells with significant atypia, marked pleomorphism, bizarre cells, mitosis, bloody, or necrotic background, CK−, Vim+, HMB45−
Kaposi sarcoma	Bloody background, clusters of spindle cells with ovoid nuclei with mostly smooth contours and finely-dispersed chromatin and 1–2 small nucleoli, HHV8+
Solitary fibrous tumor	Spindle cells and round cells in cell groups, dissociated cells and naked nuclei; CD34+
Pleomorphic/spindle cell carcinoma	Giant cells (2–10 nuclei, pleomorphic) and mononuclear cells have significant atypia, nuclear blebbing, marked pleomorphism, dyscohesive cell pattern, neutrophils within cytoplasm, bizarre cells, tumor necrosis, CK+ Vim+/−, HMB45−, S100−
Melanoma, pleomorphic	Atypical mononuclear and giant cells with significant atypia, marked pleomorphism, bizarre cells, discohesive cell pattern, giant nucleoli, nuclear inclusions, central grooving, CK− Vim+, HMB45+, S100+, Melan A+

References

1. Geisinger KR, Abdul-Karim FW. Fine needle aspiration biopsies of soft tissue tumors. In: Weiss SW, Goldblum JR, eds. *Enzinger and Weiss Soft Tissue Tumors*. 5th ed. Saint Louis: Mosby; 2008:103–118.
2. Kilpatrick SE, Ward WG, Cappellari JO, Bos GD. Fine-needle aspiration biopsy of soft tissue sarcomas. A cytomorphologic analysis with emphasis on histologic subtyping, grading, and therapeutic significance. *Ann Diagn Pathol*. 1999;3(1):48–61.
3. Handa U, Bhutani A, Mohan H, Bawa AS. Role of fine needle aspiration cytology in nonneoplastic testicular and scrotal lesions and male infertility. *Acta Cytol*. 2006;50(5):51–57.
4. Hummel P, Cangiarella JF, Cohen JM, Yang G, Waisman J, Chhieng DC. Transthoracic fine-needle aspiration biopsy of pulmonary spindle cell and mesenchymal lesions: a study of 61 cases. *Cancer*. 2001;93(3):187–198.
5. Wong NL. Fine needle aspiration cytology of pseudosarcomatous reactive proliferative lesions of soft tissue. *Acta Cytol*. 2002;46(6): 1049–1055.
6. Dodd LG, Marom EM, Dash RC, Matthews MR, McLendon RE. Fine-needle aspiration cytology of "ancient" schwannoma. *Diagn Cytopathol*. 1999;20(5):307–11.
7. Mooney EE, Layfield LJ, Dodd LG. Fine-needle aspiration of neural lesions. *Diagn Cytopathol*. 1999;20(1):1–5.
8. Domanski HA, Carlén B, Jonsson K, Mertens F, Akerman M. Distinct cytologic features of spindle cell lipoma. A cytologic-histologic study with clinical, radiologic, electron microscopic, and cytogenetic correlations. *Cancer*. 2001;93(6):381–389.
9. Agoff SN, Folpe AL, Grieco VS, Garcia RL. Spindle cell lipoma of the oral cavity. Report of a rare intramuscular case with fine needle aspiration findings. *Acta Cytol*. 2001;45(1):93–98. Review.
10. Villaschi S, Macciomei MC. Solitary fibrous tumor of the perithyroid soft tissue. Report of a case simulating a thyroid nodule. *Ann Ital Chir*. 1996;67(1):89–91.
11. Martinez V, Sissons HA. Aneurysmal bone cyst. A review of 123 cases including primary lesions and those secondary to other bone pathology. *Cancer*. 1988;61(11):2291–2304.
12. Yamamoto T, Nagira K, Akisue T, et al. Fine-needle aspiration biopsy of solid aneurysmal bone cyst in the humerus. *Diagn Cytopathol*. 2003;28(3):159–162.
13. Laforga JB, Jover A, Martínez P. Soft-tissue osteosarcoma with prominent aneurysmatic bone cyst-like features: a case report. *Diagn Cytopathol*. 2001;24(3):209–214.

14. Domanski HA, Akerman M, Rissler P, Gustafson P. Fine-needle aspiration of soft tissue leiomyosarcoma: an analysis of the most common cytologic findings and the value of ancillary techniques. *Diagn Cytopathol.* 2006;34(9):597–604.

15. Fleshman R, Mayerson J, Wakely PE Jr. Fine-needle aspiration biopsy of high-grade sarcoma: a report of 107 cases. *Cancer.* 2007;111(6):491–498.

16. Omeroglu G, Ersşahin C, Potkul RK, Booth CN. FNA diagnosis of retroperitoneal leiomyosarcoma metastasizing to the breast. *Diagn Cytopathol.* 2007;35(8):508–511.

17. Klijanienko J, Caillaud JM, Lagacé R, Vielh P. Comparative fine-needle aspiration and pathologic study of malignant fibrous histiocytoma: cytodiagnostic features of 95 tumors in 71 patients. *Diagn Cytopathol.* 2003;29(6):320–326.

18. Hirachand S, Lakhey M, Singha AK, Devkota S, Akhter J. Fine needle aspiration (FNA) of soft tissue tumours (STT. *Kathmandu Univ Med J (KUMJ).* 2007;5(3):374–377.

19. Akerman M. Fine-needle aspiration cytology of soft tissue sarcoma: benefits and limitations. *Sarcoma.* 1998;2(3-4):155–161.

20. Willén H, Akerman M, Carlén B. Fine needle aspiration (FNA) in the diagnosis of soft tissue tumours; a review of 22 years experience. *Cytopathology.* 1995;6(4):236–247.

21. Akerman M, Domanski H. *The Cytology of Soft Tissue Tumors*, vol. 16. Switzerland: Karger; 2003:83–84.

22. Silverberg S, DeLellis R, Frable W, LiVolsi V, Wick M. *Silverberg's Principles and Practice of Surgical Pathology and Cytopathology*, vol. 1. 4th ed. China: Elsevier Inc; 2006:388.

23. Siddiqui NH, Jani J. Osteosarcoma metastatic to adrenal gland diagnosed by fine-needle aspiration. *Diagn Cytopathol.* 2005;33(3):201–204.

24. Domanski HA, Akerman M. Fine-needle aspiration of primary osteosarcoma: a cytological-histological study. *Diagn Cytopathol.* 2005; 32(5):269–275.

25. Fulciniti F, Di Mattia D, Bove P, et al. Fine needle aspiration of metastatic epithelioid angiosarcoma: a report of 2 cases. *Acta Cytol.* 2008;52(5):612–618.

26. Pai MR, Upadhyaya K, Naik R, Malhotra S. Bilateral angiosarcoma breast diagnosed by fine needle aspiration cytology. *Indian J Pathol Microbiol.* 2008;51(3):421–423.

27. Gamborino E, Carrilho C, Ferro J, et al. Fine-needle aspiration diagnosis of Kaposi's sarcoma in a developing country. *Diagn Cytopathol.* 2000;23:322–325.

28. Molina CP, Putegnat BB, Logroño R. Fine-needle aspiration cytology and core biopsy of malignant peripheral nerve sheath tumor of the uterus: a case report. *Diagn Cytopathol.* 2001;24(5):347–351.

29. Dodd LG, Scully S, Layfield LJ. Fine-needle aspiration of epithelioid malignant peripheral nerve sheath tumor (epithelioid malignant schwannoma). *Diagn Cytopathol.* 1997;17(3):200–204.
30. Bardarov S, Michael CW, Lucas D, Pang Y, Pu RT. Fine-needle aspiration biopsy of metastatic malignant melanoma resembling a malignant peripheral nerve sheath tumor. *Diagn Cytopathol.* 2008;36(10):754–757.
31. Piao Y, Guo M, Gong Y. Diagnostic challenges of metastatic spindle cell melanoma on fine-needle aspiration specimens. *Cancer.* 2008;114(2):94–101.
32. Morgan MB, Purohit C, Anglin TR. Immunohistochemical distinction of cutaneous spindle cell carcinoma. *Am J Dermatopathol.* 2008;30(3):228–232.
33. Matthai SM, Kini U. Aspiration cytology of sarcomatoid carcinoma of the breast: report of a case with cystic change. *Diagn Cytopathol.* 2004;31(1):10–13.

4
Cytopathology of Soft Tissue and Bone Lesions Containing Giant Cells

There are varieties of soft tissue and bone lesions that are characterized by a prominence of multinucleated giant cells. The giant cells can be reactive or tumorous. The presence of bland-appearing giant cell nuclei does not indicate benign lesions, since certain high-grade malignancies such as giant-rich osteosarcoma and osteoclast-like giant cell pleomorphic carcinoma may contain reactive osteoclastic giant cells that appear cytologically bland.[1,2] However, the presence of giant cells with significant nuclear atypia only seen in malignant conditions. The differential diagnoses of soft tissue and bone with prominence giant cells include[1-3] benign lesions, low-grade malignant tumors, and high-grade malignant tumors (see Table 4.1). The benign conditions include giant cell tumor of tendon sheath, giant-cell reparative granuloma, fat necrosis, pigmented villonodular synovitis, and brown tumor of hyperparathyroidism. The low-grade malignant tumors include giant cell tumor of bone, soft tissue giant cell tumor of low malignant potential, and myxoid low-grade malignant fibrous histiocytoma (MFH). The high-grade malignant tumors include chondroblastoma, anaplastic MFH, giant cell-rich osteosarcoma, pleomorphic high-grade sarcoma (rhabdomyosarcoma, liposarcoma, and leiomyosarcoma), giant cell carcinoma, malignant melanoma, and anaplastic large cell lymphoma (see Table 4.1).

W.E. Khalbuss and A.V. Parwani, *Cytopathology of Soft Tissue and Bone Lesions*, Essentials in Cytopathology 9, DOI 10.1007/978-1-4419-6499-1_4, © Springer Science+Business Media, LLC 2011

TABLE 4.1. The differential diagnosis of soft tissue and bone tumors with giant cells.

Benign	Malignant
• Giant cell tumor of tendon sheath/pigmented villonodular synovitis	• Giant cell tumor of bone
• Myositis ossificans/nodular fasciitis	• Soft tissue giant cell tumor of low malignant potential
• Giant-cell reparative granuloma	• Sarcomas/pleomorphic sarcoma: 　◦ Malignant fibrous histiocytoma (MFH) 　◦ Rhabdomyosarcoma 　◦ Liposarcoma 　◦ Leiomyosarcoma 　◦ Giant cell-rich osteosarcoma
• Nodular tenosynovitis/ossifying myositis	• Metastatic giant cell carcinoma • Malignant melanoma • Anaplastic large cell lymphoma

Giant Cell Tumor of Tendon Sheath/Pigmented Villonodular Synovitis[4–9] (Fig. 4.1)

- Also known as: tenosynovitis, giant cell tumor of tendon sheath.
- Locally aggressive proliferative disorder of the synovial lining of the joints
- Localized or diffuse nodular thickening of the synovial membrane.
- Proliferation of mononuclear histiocytes and giant cells.
- Affects major joints including fingers, knee, ankle, hip, and shoulder.
- It is usually occurs in the flexor tendon sheath.
- The bone underlying the lesion may be eroded giving the impression of an osseous tumor.

Cytomorphology of Giant Cell Tumor of Tendon Sheath

- Predominantly mononuclear, with histiocytoid cells in single and clusters or in papillary configuration.
- Coarse, refractile, golden brown crystals of hemosiderin within the cells.

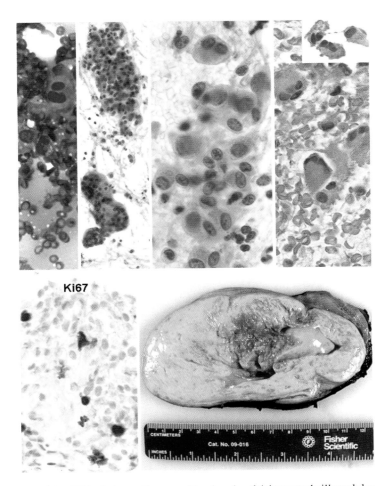

Fig. 4.1. FNA of giant cell tumor of tendon sheath/pigmented villonodular synovitis (DQ, *left upper* ×400; Pap stain *middle* ×100 and 400, and cell block *right* ×400, *left lower*, Ki67 immunostain ×200, and *lower right* gross photograph of the subsequent excisional biopsy of the mass). The patient is a 48-year-old female who presented with large thigh mass. The smears are hypocellular with predominance of mononuclear, histiocytoid cells, and giant cells. The histiocytoid cells arranged singly and in clusters with some showing papillary configuration. The multinucleated giant cells show uniformly sized nuclei similar to those of mononuclear cells. Immunostain of Ki67 shows low proliferative index. The subsequent excisional biopsy shows 12-cm well-circumscribed mass and diagnosis of villonodular synovitis was confirmed.

- Multinucleated giant cells with uniformly sized, bland-appearing nuclei (similar to mononuclear cells).
- Intranuclear inclusions can be seen.
- Inflammatory cells are scanty.

Ancillary Studies

Prussian blue+; Vimentin+, CD68+, Calponin+; Cytokeratin−, S100−, and CD34−, Ki67 (low index).

Differential Diagnosis

- Soft tissue giant cell tumor of low malignant potential (less heterogeneous population of cells, no prominent stromal hyalinization), melanoma,
- Sarcomas.

Giant Cell Tumor of Bone[10,11] (Figs. 4.2 and 4.3)

- Also known as osteoclastoma
- 4% of all primary bone tumors.
- Ages 20–40 years; more common in Asian countries
- Knee is common site (distal femur, proximal tibia), distal radius, and sacrum.
- It is a low-grade malignancy
- Can metastasize to lung or lymph nodes (1–2%)
- 1/3 have focal deposition of osteoid or bone
- It may have aneurysmal bone cyst (ABC) component, foam cells with spindling of mononuclear cells; no chondroid differentiation, no atypia

Cytomorphology of Giant Cell Tumor of Bone

- Mononuclear cells resembling macrophages, intermingled with giant multinucleated cells (10–50 nuclei) with similar nuclei (bland-appearing) as stromal cells, resembling osteoclasts.
- Histiocytes, large numbers of osteoclast-like giant cells in a background of epithelioid to spindle-shaped mononuclear cells.
- Stromal cells are mononuclear, resemble macrophages.

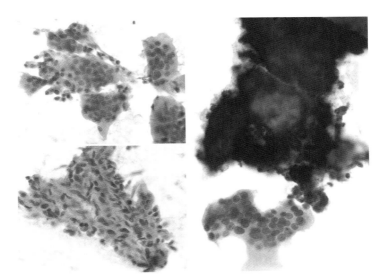

FIG. 4.2. FNA of giant cell tumor of bone. The patient was 15-year-old male who presented with 4-cm lytic tibial mass. The smears contain mononuclear stromal cells and are intimately associated with numerous multinucleated giant cells. The nuclei in both mononuclear and giant cells are similar, showing bland oval nuclei with fine chromatin and small nucleoli. Some of the giant cells contain more than 50 nuclei. Osteoid tissue is also present. (Pap stain x200).

- Necrosis, hemorrhage, hemosiderin, reactive bone; mitotic figures (typical).
- Typically pulmonary implants are solitary lesions characterized by a very slow growth rate and a non-aggressive clinical course.

Ancillary Studies

Lysozyme+, alpha-1-antitrypsin+, alpha-1-antichymotrypsin+, calcitonin+, ER+, and metalloproteinases+.

Differential Diagnosis

- Brown tumor of hyperthyroidism,
- Giant cell granuloma,
- Pigmented villonodular synovitis,

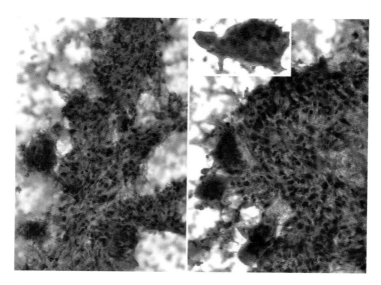

FIG. 4.3. FNA of lung metastasis of giant cell tumor of bone. The patient was a 34-year-old-female who had history of spinal giant cell tumor (T9) of bone 3 years prior, and then presented with a lung mass. FNA of lung mass shows mononuclear stromal cells that are intimately associated with numerous multinucleated giant cells. The nuclei in both mononuclear and giant cells are similar and bland, and resemble the previously resected giant cell tumor 3 years ago. (Pap stain, *left* ×200, *right* ×400) The lung pulmonary implant was a solitary lesion, but extended into the ribs. These tumor implants are usually very slow growing and show non-aggressive clinical course.

- Chondroblastoma,
- ABC;
- Osteosarcoma, and Langerhans cell histiocytosis.

Aneurysmal Bone Cyst[12-14] (Fig. 4.4)

- Uncommon blowout distension of cortical bony contour lesion.
- Radiologically: extensive ballooning of the bone contour (soap bubble appearance).
- Usually young, ages 1–20 years (80%) with recurrence in 20%
- Metaphysis of posterior vertebrae (often multiple), flat bones, shaft of long bones; May also be secondary to trauma or arise

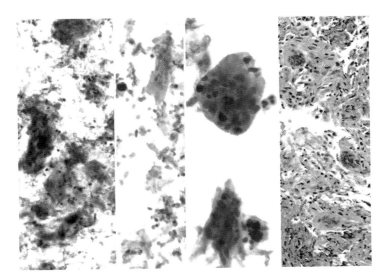

FIG. 4.4. FNA of aneurysmal bone cyst: Clusters of osteoclast-like multinucleated giant cells with loose spindly stroma to cellular stroma. The cell block shows fragments of bland-appearing fibroconnective tissue with fibroblasts, myofibroblasts; histiocytes, and giant cells without endothelium; no malignant osteoid, no atypia. (*Left* to *right*, Pap stain ×200, ×200, ×400, H&E cell block, ×200) The excisional biopsy of this lesion showed aneurysmal bone cyst with infarction.

  in preexisting bone lesion (giant cell tumor, chondroblastoma, fibrous dysplasia)
- Benign; grows rapidly, multiloculated locally aggressive cystic neoplasm.
- Expanding osteolytic lesion of blood-filled spaces of variable size separated by connective tissue septa with osteoclast giant cells, and variable reactive bone
- Rarely transforms to osteosarcoma

Cytomorphology of Aneurysmal Bone Cyst

- Fragments of fibroconnective tissue
- Cysts and septa lined by fibroblasts, myofibroblasts and histiocytes but not endothelium

- Clusters of osteoclast-like multinucleated giant cells with loose spindly stroma to cellular stroma
- Reactive woven bone, degenerated calcifying fibromyxoid tissue; variable mitotic figures and hemosiderin; no malignant osteoid, no atypia Ancillary Studies

Molecular: Abnormalities of 17p13.2 loci in 63%.

Differential Diagnosis

- Solitary bone cyst,
- Giant cell tumor (lacks fibroblastic cells), hemangioma,
- Telangiectatic osteosarcoma (more atypia),
- Giant cell reparative granuloma (if in jaw),
- Low-grade osteosarcoma (hypocellular).

Myelolipoma[15] (Fig. 4.5)

- Rare tumor-like growth of bone marrow elements mixed with mature fat.
- Soft tissue/extraadrenal sites such as presacral are rare.
- Usually an incidental finding at autopsy (0.1–0.2%) or CT/ MRI.
- Not associated with hematologic disorders (non-functioning lesion).
- Most patients are obese adults (mean age 50 years).
- May have areas of fibromyxoid degeneration resembling low-grade fibromyxoid sarcomas.
- May be metaplastic change in reticuloendothelial cells of blood capillaries in response to necrosis, infection, or stress.

Cytomorphology of Myelolipoma

- Mature islands of hematopoietic precursor cells and mature fat.
- The hematopoietic cells contain mixture of trilineage bone marrow elements and megakaryocytes.
- Megakaryocytes may be prominent and display cytological atypia.
- Hemorrhage, necrosis, calcification and cyst formation in large tumors.

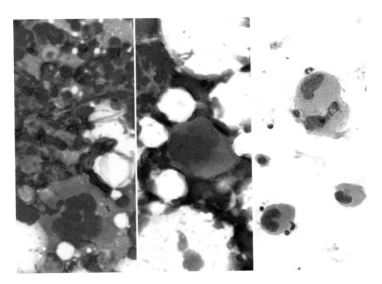

FIG. 4.5. FNA of Myelolipoma presented as sacral mass. The smears (DQ and Pap stained, ×400) show admixture of adipose tissue and hematopoietic bone marrow elements with prominence of megakaryocytes. The multinucleation with some cytological nuclear atypia in megakaryocytes mimics liposarcoma. However, the presence of numerous bone marrow elements should alert to this lesion.

Differential Diagnosis

- Liposarcoma,
- Extramedullary hematopoietic tumors.

Subcutaneous Fat Necrosis[16–18] (Fig. 4.6)

- It is common in all ages including newborn.
- Degeneration of adipose tissue caused by trauma, inflammation, or malignancy.
- It may result in cyst formation, hemorrhage, calcification, or fibrosis.

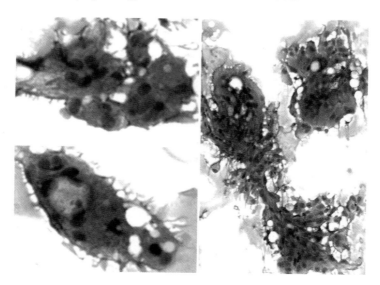

FIG. 4.6. FNA of subcutaneous fat necrosis. Adipose tissue lesion with numerous lipid-laden foam cells, lipid-laden large, foreign-body giant cells, and epithelioid cells. (Pap stain, both *left* ×400, *right* ×200)

- Common sites are subcutaneous tissue of the buttock or abdomen of obese persons.
- Resemble adipose tissue tumors and may be deep-seated.

Cytomorphology of Fat Necrosis

- Variable numbers of foam cells, giant cells, and elongated epithelioid cells with dark nuclei and lipid-laden and hemosiderin-laden macrophages.
- The large, foreign-body giant cells may show intracytoplasmic inclusions.
- Leukocytes, cholesterol crystals, and calcification may also be seen.

Ancillary Studies

CD68+, S100+, CK–

Differential Diagnosis

- Granulomatous inflammation,
- Lipomatous tumors

Nodular Fasciitis and Myositis Ossificans[16]
(Fig. 4.7)

- Reparative pseudosarcomatous lesions
- Affects healthy, active adolescents with history of trauma
- May arise in the subcutis and musculature of the upper and lower extremities
- Presents as painless, well-demarcated mass with rapid growth

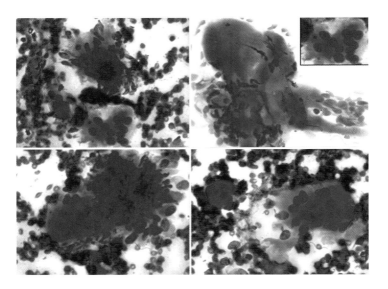

FIG. 4.7. FNA of myositis ossificans with prominence of giant cells presented as large arm mass from 69-year-old male (DQ stain, all ×400). The smears show predominance of bland-appearing spindle cells and giant cells with bland-appearing nuclei. The background is edematous/myxoid. Numerous plasmacytoid and polygonal multinucleated osteoclast-type of cells are seen. Muscle tissue is also present (*upper right*). The subsequent excisional biopsy confirmed the diagnosis of myositis ossificans.

Cytomorphology of Nodular Fasciitis & Myositis Ossificans

- Cytology shows mixed pattern of high cellularity, low cellularity, spindle cells, muscle cells, osteoblasts, giant cells, myxoid areas, edematous areas, and occasional bone tissue.
- The predominant cell type is spindle cells and/or giant cells.
- Granular, fibrillar, and myxoid background may be prominent.
- Plasmacytoid or polygonal osteoblasts and multinucleated osteoclasts may be prominent in some cases.
- No osteoid or chondroid, and no cytological atypia.

Ancillary Studies

Vimentin+, MSA (+), calponin (+), Cytokeratin (−), S100 (−), and CD34 (−), Ki67 (low index)

Differential Diagnosis

- Osteosarcoma,
- Giant cell tumor

Sarcomas with Giant Cell/Pleomorphic Morphology[19–23] (Figs. 4.8–4.10)

There are several sarcomas that present with giant cell morphology, such as myxoid fibrosarcoma, pleomorphic sarcomas (rhabdomyosarcoma, leiomyosarcoma, liposarcoma, chondrosarcoma, giant cell-rich osteosarcoma).

Cytomorphology of Sarcomas with Giant Cells

- Smears usually very cellular with pleomorphic spindle cell population.
- Mononucleated, binucleated, and multinucleated cells with marked pleomorphism.
- Marked nuclear atypia/abnormalities with coarse chromatin, macronucleoli.
- The predominant cell type is spindle cells and/or giant cells.

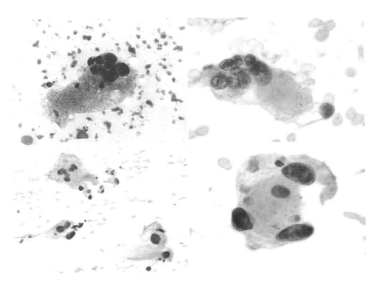

F<small>IG</small>. 4.8.   FNA of high-grade sarcoma. The patient was a 77-year-old male who had history of high-grade sarcoma of left arm. He presented with new arm nodule. The smears (DQ stained *upper left* ×400, and Pap-stained smears *lower left* ×200, and *right*, ×400) showed markedly pleomorphic cells showing marked nuclear atypia and necrotic background consistent with recurrent high-grade sarcoma.

- Granular, fibrillar, myxoid, or necrotic background may be prominent.
- Bizarre cells and mitoses.

Ancillary Studies

Vimentin+, MSA (+), Calponin (+), Myogenin (leiomyosarcoma and rhabdomyosarcoma), S100 (in liposarcoma and MPNST); CD68 (in MFH); Osteonectin+ (in osteosarcoma); Ki67+; cytokeratin (−), CD34 (−).

Differential Diagnosis

- Giant cell carcinoma,
- Malignant melanoma,
- Anaplastic lymphoma.

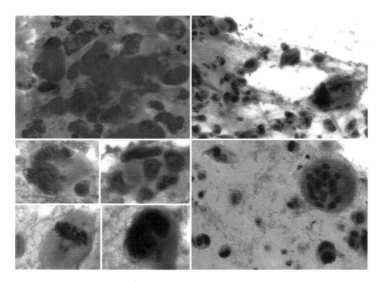

Fig. 4.9. FNA of pleomorphic rhabdomyosarcoma. The patient is a 59-year-old male who presented with 8-cm elbow mass. The smears (DQ stained *upper left*, ×400, and Pap-stained *upper right* ×200, *Lower, left and right* ×400), showed markedly pleomorphic atypical cells arranged haphazardly in sheets and in single arrangement. The individual cells are round or polygonal with large, hyperchromatic nuclei, and deeply eosinophilic cytoplasm. The nuclei are characterized by thickened nuclear membranes associated with indentations (*left lower*). The immunostain in this case on cell block material showed positive nuclear staining for myogenin confirming diagnosis of pleomorphic rhabdomyosarcoma.

Metastatic Giant Cell Carcinoma of Lung, Pancreas,[2] Thyroid, or Kidney (Fig. 4.11)

- History of carcinoma in most cases
- Highly cellular specimen
- Dispersed cell pattern
- Markedly pleomorphic cells with frequent of giant cells
- Nuclei with irregular, coarse and clumped chromatin, and parachromatin clearing
- Single or multiple prominent nucleoli
- Intranuclear inclusions
- Mitosis and necrosis

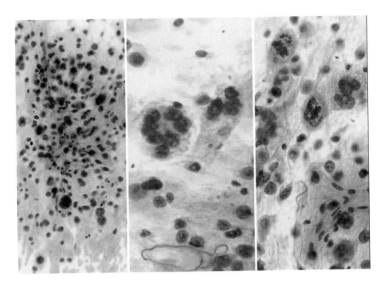

FIG. 4.10. FNA of malignant fibrous histiocytoma, myxoid type. The smears (Pap stained) are abundantly cellular and demonstrate single and loosely cohesive clusters of highly atypical spindle and polygonal-round cells in an abundant mucinous background. The cells display pleomorphism, and marked anisokaryosis. Nuclei have an irregular, with coarse chromatin distribution. Admixed are large multinucleated giant cells and histiocyte-like cells having increased amounts of vacuolated cytoplasm. Also seen is high number of mitotic figures including atypical mitoses. Numerous large pleomorphic cells are also seen. The subsequent histological biopsy confirms malignant fibrous histiocytoma, myxoid type. (Pap stain, *left* ×200, *middle* & *right* ×400)

Ancillary Studies

Vimentin−, CK+; May be TTF-1+, Thyroglobin+, or CA19.9+ depending upon the primary tumor

Differential Diagnosis

- Pleomorphic sarcoma,
- Malignant melanoma,
- Anaplastic lymphoma

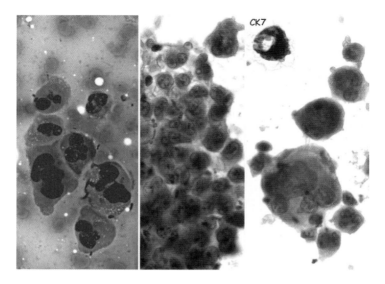

FIG. 4.11.   FNA of metastatic giant cell carcinoma of the lung. Patient with history of spinal soft tissue mass diagnosed as giant cell tumor of the bone, presented with lung mass. The smears (DQ stained, *left* ×600, and Pap stained, *right* ×400 and ×600) are highly cellular with predominance of dispersed cell pattern. The cells are markedly pleomorphic cells with numerous giant cells showing markedly abnormal nuclei (irregular, coarse and clumped chromatin, parachromatin clearing, prominent nucleoli). Mitosis and necrosis are also present. The cytokeratin 7 (CK7) was positive in giant cells (*inset*).

Metastatic Malignant Melanoma[24,25] (Fig. 4.12)

- History of melanoma in most cases
- Highly cellular smear, dispersed cell pattern
- Cytomorphology of Metastatic Melanoma
- Marked variation in size and shape
- Oval, triangular, plasmacytoid, polygonal, spindle shape, caudate forms
- Well-defined cell border, clear or dusty cytoplasm
- Variable N/C ratio
- Binucleation, multinucleate with bizarre forms
- Large irregular cherry-red macronucleoli or multiple micronucleoli

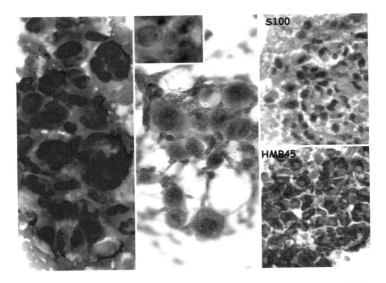

F<small>IG</small>. 4.12. FNA of malignant melanoma with giant cell features. The patient is a 57-year-old male who presented with chest wall mass. The smears (DQ, *left* ×400 and Pap stained, *middle* ×400) showed markedly pleomorphic, dyscohesive cell pattern (best seen in Pap-stained smear); an intranuclear inclusion is noted (*inset*). Immunostain study showed positive staining for S100 and HMB45 (*right* ×200) confirming diagnosis of malignant melanoma.

- Intranuclear cytoplasmic inclusions
- Mitotic figures

Ancillary Studies

S100+, HMB45+, Melan A+, CK−

Differential Diagnosis

- Pleomorphic sarcoma,
- Giant cell carcinoma,
- Anaplastic lymphoma

Anaplastic Large Cell Lymphoma Involving Soft Tissue or Bone[26,27] (Fig. 4.13)

- High-grade T-cell malignancy, usually history is present in most cases.
- Comprises 5% of all non-Hodgkin lymphoma (NHL)
- More in males, 3:2; and may arise in HIV-positive patients.
- Two forms: primary cutaneous form and systemic form
- Prognosis depends on anaplastic lymphoma kinase (ALK) expression (ALK-positive 5-year survival rate 70–80%; and ALK-negative 5-year survival rate 15–30%).

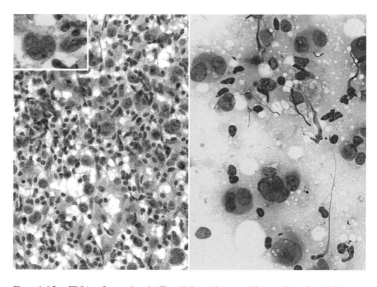

FIG. 4.13. FNA of anaplastic T-cell lymphoma. The patient is a 20-year-old male who presented with chest wall mass. The smears (Pap and DQ stained, ×200 and ×400, respectively) showed high cellular aspirates with sheets of malignant cells, some showing large, bizarre, markedly pleomorphic cells with moderatly dense basophilic cytoplasm and large, angulated, eccentrically placed nuclei. Coarse granular chromatin with prominent nucleoli also noted (see *inset*). The background of heterogeneous cells, lymphocytes and few lymphoglandular bodies also seen.

Cytomorphology of ALCL

- Abundantly cellular aspirates with sheets of malignant lymphoid cells
- Large, bizarre, markedly pleomorphic cells
- Moderate amounts of dense basophilic cytoplasm
- Large, angulated, eccentrically placed nuclei
- Numerous multi-lobated nuclei, and binucleated cells are seen
- Scattered mitotic figures and apoptotic bodies are present
- Coarse granular chromatin with prominent nucleoli
- Some appear immunoblast-like
- Background of heterogeneous cells: Lymphocytes, plasma cells, and histiocytes
- Lymphoglandular bodies may be sparse

Ancillary Studies

T-cell phenotype, CD3+, CD4+, CD8−; CD30 (75%) ALK, monoclonal rearrangement of the *TCR* gene, and often t(2;5) translocation in systemic form.

Differential Diagnosis

- Hodgkin disease,
- Granulocytic sarcoma,
- Pleomorphic sarcoma, malignant melanoma,
- Giant cell carcinoma.

Summary

There are varieties of soft tissue and bone lesions that are characterized by giant cell morphology including reactive, benign, and malignant neoplasms. The malignant neoplasms with giant cell morphology can be mesenchymal/sarcomas, carcinomas, melanomas, and anaplastic lymphomas. The key features to be examined are the number of nuclei in giant cells, presence of cytological atypia and pleomorphism in giant cells, the mononuclear cell morphology, and the background morphology (See Table 4.2). Ancillary studies are a crucial particularly for the initial diagnosis.

TABLE 4.2. FNA of giant cell-containing lesions affecting soft tissue and bone.

Entity	Key cytological features
Nodular fasciitis	Giant cells (2–10 nuclei, bland) and mononuclear cells have no atypia, uniform nuclei, mixed cell pattern
Fat necrosis/ granulomas	Foreign-body giant cells (2–10 nuclei, bland) and lipophages with no atypia, epithelioid cell, bloody or necrotic background; PMNs and lymphocytes
Giant cell tumor of tendon sheath	Giant cells (3–50 nuclei) and mononuclear cells have no atypia; uniform nuclei; hemosiderin pigments; xanthocyte, clean or granular debris background
Giant cell tumor of bone	Giant cells (10–100 nuclei) and mononuclear cells have no atypia; uniform nuclei; no hemosiderin pigments, clean or bloody background
Sarcoma, pleomorphic	Giant cells (10–20 nuclei, pleomorphic); mononuclear cells have significant atypia and marked pleomorphism, bizarre cells, bloody or necrotic background, CK−, Vim+, HMB45−
Giant-cell-rich osteosarcoma	Giant cells (2–10 nuclei, bland, uniform, osteoclastic) and mononuclear cells have significant atypia and marked pleomorphism, bizarre cells, bloody or necrotic background, CK−, Vim+, HMB45−, osteonectin+
Melanoma, pleomorphic	Giant cells (2–10 nuclei, pleomorphic) and mononuclear cells have significant atypia, marked pleomorphism, bizarre cells, discohesive cell pattern, giant nucleoli, nuclear inclusions, central grooving, CK− Vim+, HMB45+, S100+, Melan A+
Giant cell carcinoma	Giant cells (2–10 nuclei, pleomorphic) and mononuclear cells have significant atypia, nuclear blebbing, marked pleomorphism, dyscohesive cell pattern, neutrophils within cytoplasm, bizarre cells, tumor necrosis, CK+ Vim+/−, HMB45−, S100−
Anaplastic lymphoma	Giant cells (2–10 nuclei, pleomorphic) and mononuclear cells have significant atypia, marked pleomorphism, dyscohesive cell pattern, bizarre cells, tumor necrosis, no significant reactive lymphocytes, CK− Vim+, HMB45−, S100−, CD45+, CD30+, EMA+/−, CD15+/−

References

1. O'Connell JX, Wehrli BM, Nielsen GP, Rosenberg AE. Giant cell tumors of soft tissue: a clinicopathologic study of 18 benign and malignant tumors. *Am J Surg Pathol*. 2000;24(3):386–395.
2. Layfield LJ, Bentz J. Giant-cell containing neoplasms of the pancreas: an aspiration cytology study. *Diagn Cytopathol*. 2008;36(4):238–244.

3. Akerman M, Domanski H. *The Cytology of Soft Tissue Tumors*, vol. 16. Switzerland: Karger; 2003:83–84.

4. Gangane N, Anshu, Shivkumar VB, Sharma SM. Intranuclear inclusions in a case of pigmented villonodular synovitis of the ankle. *Diagn Cytopathol*. 2003;29(6):349–351.

5. Oliveira AM, DeiTos AP, Fletcher CD, Nascimento AG. Primary giant cell tumor of soft tissues: a study of 22 cases. *Am J Surg Pathol*. 2000;24(2):248–256.

6. Dawisikiba S, Eriksson L, Elner A, Johansen CC, Hansson L-G, Westeon P-L. Diffuse pigmented villonodular synovitis of the temporomandibular joint diagnosed by fine needle aspiration cytology. *Diagn Cytopathol*. 1989;5:301–304.

7. Chhieng DC, Boguniewicz A, McKenna BJ. Pigmented villonodular synovitis: report of a case with diagnostic synovial fluid cytologic

8. Iyer VK, Kapila K, Verma K. Fine-needle aspiration cytology of giant cell tumor of tendon sheath. *Diagn Cytopathol*. 2003;29(2):105–110.

9. Agarwal PK, Gupta M, Srivastava A, Agarwal S. Cytomorphology of giant cell tumor of tendon sheath. A report of two cases. *Acta Cytol*. 1997;41(2):587–589.

10. Sneige N, Ayala AG, Carrasco CH, Murray J, Raymond AK. Giant cell tumor of bone. A cytologic study of 24 cases. *Diagn Cytopathol*. 1985;1(2):111–117.

11. Haque AU, Moatasim A. Giant cell tumor of bone: a neoplasm or a reactive condition? *Int J Clin Exp Pathol*. 2008;1(6):489–501.

12. Martinez V, Sissons HA. Aneurysmal bone cyst. A review of 123 cases including primary lesions and those secondary to other bone pathology. *Cancer*. 1988;61(11):2291–2304.

13. Yamamoto T, Nagira K, Akisue T, et al. Fine-needle aspiration biopsy of solid aneurysmal bone cyst in the humerus. *Diagn Cytopathol*. 2003;28(3):159–162.

14. Laforga JB, Jover A, Martínez P. Soft-tissue osteosarcoma with prominent aneurysmatic bone cyst-like features: a case report. *Diagn Cytopathol*. 2001;24(3):209–214.

15. Settakorn J, Sirivanichai C, Rangdaeng S, Chaiwun B. Fine-needle aspiration cytology of adrenal myelolipoma: case report and review of the literature. *Diagn Cytopathol*. 1999;21(6):409–412.

16. Wong NL. Fine needle aspiration cytology of pseudosarcomatous reactive proliferative lesions of soft tissue. *Acta Cytol*. 2002;46(6):1049–1055.

17. Canteli B, Saez F, de los Ríos A, Alvarez C. Fat necrosis. *Skeletal Radiol*. 1996;25(3):305–307.

18. Tsai TS, Evans HA, Donnelly LF, Bisset GS 3rd, Emery KH. Fat necrosis after trauma: a benign cause of palpable lumps in children. *AJR Am J Roentgenol*. 1997;169(6):1623–1626.

19. Klijanienko J, Caillaud JM, Orbach D, et al. Cyto-histological correlations in primary, recurrent and metastatic rhabdomyosarcoma: the institut Curie's experience. *Diagn Cytopathol.* 2007;35(8):482–487.

20. Klijanienko J, Caillaud JM, Lagacé R. Fine-needle aspiration of primary and recurrent benign fibrous histiocytoma: classic, aneurysmal, and myxoid variants. *Diagn Cytopathol.* 2004;31(6):387–391.

21. Domanski HA, Akerman M, Rissler P, Gustafson P. Fine-needle aspiration of soft tissue leiomyosarcoma: an analysis of the most common cytologic findings and the value of ancillary techniques. *Diagn Cytopathol.* 2006;34(9):597–604.

22. Klijanienko J, Caillaud JM, Lagacé R, et al. Comparative fine-needle aspiration and pathologic study of malignant fibrous histiocytoma: cytodiagnostic features of 95 tumors in 71 patients. *Diagn Cytopathol.* 2003;29(6):320–326.

23. Skoog L, Pereira ST, Tani E. Fine-needle aspiration cytology and immunocytochemistry of soft-tissue tumors and osteo/chondrosarcomas of the head and neck. *Diagn Cytopathol.* 1999;20(3):131–136.

24. Piao Y, Guo M, Gong Y. Diagnostic challenges of metastatic spindle cell melanoma on fine-needle aspiration specimens. *Diagn Cytopathol.* 1999;20(3):131–136.

25. Piao Y, Guo M, Gong Y. Diagnostic challenges of metastatic spindle cell melanoma on fine-needle aspiration specimens. *Cancer.* 2008;114(2):94–101.

26. Kim SE, Kim SH, Lim BJ, Hong SW, Yang WI. Fine needle aspiration cytology of small cell variant of anaplastic large cell lymphoma. A case report. *Acta Cytol.* 2004;48(2):254–258.

27. Medeiros LJ, Elenitoba-Johnson KS. Anaplastic Large Cell Lymphoma. *Am J Clin Pathol.* 2007;127(5):707–722.

5
Cytopathology of Myxoid Soft Tissue Lesions

Myxoid soft tissue lesions are a group of lesions that are distinguished by their unique and consistent ability to produce an overwhelming abundance of myxoid ground substance along with the proliferating cells that constitute the lesion. The myxoid material is composed of sulfated and nonsulfated glycosaminoglycans. It appears on H&E sections as a thin amorphous semitransparent or grey substance. Special stains such as alcian blue can confirm its presence and only sulfated glycosaminoglycans (chondroid substance) will be positive after treatment by hyaluronidase.

Most soft tissue tumors and pseudotumors may show limited myxoid areas. However, significant myxoid background provides certain differential diagnoses which help in the work-up of those lesions. The differential diagnosis of myxoid soft tissue lesions includes non-neoplastic lesions such as ganglion and nodular fasciitis, benign neoplasms such as myxoma, myxoid neurilemoma, myxoid neurofibroma, spindle cell lipoma with myxoid changes, and malignant lesions such as myxoid liposarcoma, myxoid chondrosarcoma, myxofibrosarcoma/myxoid malignant fibrous histiocytoma, chordoma, low-grade fibromyxoid sarcoma, and metastatic mucinous carcinoma (see Table 5.1). Grossly, these lesions have a variable gelatinous quality.

When cytologic aspirate smears contain an abundance of myxoid material, a variety of entities enter the differential diagnosis. The majority of neoplasms fall into the category of soft tissue

W.E. Khalbuss and A.V. Parwani, *Cytopathology of Soft Tissue and Bone Lesions*, Essentials in Cytopathology 9,
DOI 10.1007/978-1-4419-6499-1_5,
© Springer Science+Business Media, LLC 2011

TABLE 5.1. The differential diagnosis of myxoid soft tissue tumors and pseudotumor.

Benign	Malignant
Most common	
Ganglion	Myxoid liposarcoma
Nodular fasciitis	Myxofibrosarcoma/myxoid MFH
Myxoma	Myxoid chondrosarcoma
Myxoid neurilemoma/neurofibroma	Chordoma
Spindle cell lipoma	Low-grade fibromyxoid sarcoma
	Metastatic carcinoma (mucinous)
Rare	
Desmoid tumor	Leiomyosarcoma
Chondroma	Synovial sarcoma
Solitary fibrous tumor	MPNST
	DFSP

neoplasms with myxoid features. However, there are also a variety of non-neoplastic changes that we have seen on aspirates of soft tissue lesions that may mimic myxoid soft tissue neoplasms. One of the most striking examples was myxoid degeneration of the soft tissue surrounding a lymphoma, which was suspicious for myxoid liposarcoma on immediate assessment. Thus, the diagnostic approach to these lesions involves immunohistochemical stains and molecular analysis, in conjunction with the cytomorphology, due to the cytomorphologic overlap in many of these entities.

The key distinguishing features that allow one to make a specific diagnosis and exclude other entities in the differential include: cellularity, cytology, vascularity, nuclear atypia, and pleomorphism. Immunohistochemical stains may help in a subset of cases to better characterize the type of cells present. Finally, the molecular studies, including FISH studies, really enable one to make a definitive diagnosis due to the characteristic translocations seen in a subset of these lesions.[1,2]

Nodular Fasciitis with Myxoid Changes (Figs. 5.1 and 5.2)

- Relatively common soft tissue tumor.
- A rapidly enlarging mass in adults, third to fourth decade.

- Mimics sarcoma, synonymous with pseudosarcomatous and infiltrative fasciitis.
- Occasionally is associated with trauma in 10–15%.
- The most common location is the forearm, but it has been described in a variety of locations, including the chest, back, and head and neck region.
- Subtypes are based on the location of the lesion.
- Subcutaneous (most common), intramuscular, and fascial.
- The lesion can regress spontaneously, but may be removed due to the concern for a neoplasm.

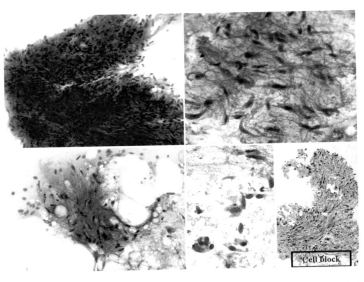

FIG. 5.1. Nodular fasciitis with myxoid changes (Pap-stained smears, *left upper* ×100, *left lower* ×200, *right upper* ×400, *middle lower* ×300, and Cell block H&E stained ×100) presented as forearm mass from 58-year-old female. The smears are hypercellular with cells, predominantly spindle, and in dense aggregates mimicking sarcoma (pseudosarcoma). Several cell types are seen including spindle, stellate fibroblasts, and polygonal. These cells mimic ganglion cells (*lower right*), and inflammatory cells. The nuclei are relatively uniform with finely granular chromatin and smooth nuclear contours. Pale blue myxoid material and granular background are readily seen in all smears in this case. No mitotic figures, no necrotic debris, and no intranuclear inclusions.

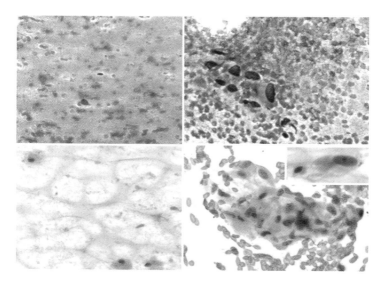

FIG. 5.2. Nodular fasciitis with myxoid changes (DQ, *upper* left ×100, upper right ×400; and Pap-stained smears, *lower* left ×300, right ×400) presented as scapular mass from 37-year-old female. The smears are hypocellular with cells in dispersed forms and small aggregate. The cells mainly spindle having a small to moderate amount of pale staining cytoplasm. The nuclei are relatively uniform with finely granular chromatin and smooth nuclear contours. Rare cell shows enlarged nucleus (*inset, lower right*). Few inflammatory cells are present. Metachromatic-staining myxoid material and granular background (more seen in DQ stain (*upper figures*). No mitotic figures, no necrotic debris, and no intranuclear inclusions. This is hypocellular nodular fasciitis that mimics myxoma.

Histological Features

- The typical histologic features include tissue culture-like fibroblasts with abundant mitoses, arranged in short bundles within a variably myxoid matrix.
- Frequently considered to be a pseudosarcoma due to its rapid growth and high mitotic activity which makes it difficult to distinguish from a spindle cell sarcoma.

Cytomorphology of Nodular Faciitis with Myxoid Changes[3]

- Hypercellular or hypocellular smears with mixed morphological pattern with myxoid and edematous background intermixed with inflammatory cells.
- The proliferating cells are a mixture (spindle, stellate fibroblasts, polygonal mimic ganglion cells, and inflammatory cells). However, they are mainly spindle with dense fields and with overlapping cells.
- The spindle shapes have a small to moderate amount of pale staining cytoplasm.
- Nuclei in relatively uniform sizes and shape, oval/elongated/finely granular chromatin and smooth or curved nuclear contours.
- Rare cell with an enlarged nucleus.
- Nucleoli are generally inconspicuous; occasionally, small nucleoli can be seen.
- Inflammatory cells (lymphocytes), extravasated red blood cells, occasional giant cells, a minor population of cells with polygonal, stellate features.
- Metachromatic-staining myxoid material and occasional granular background.
- Micro fragments of collagenous stroma are common (varied in size and shape, ranging from a few strands of collagen to very large dense fragments).
- Occasionally, cells are embedded within the larger fragments.
- No or rare mitotic figures, no necrotic debris, and no intranuclear inclusions.
- Long-standing lesions can have more of a fibrotic or hyalinized appearance, whereas the lesions with a more myxoid appearance are usually new or recent lesions. Therefore, older lesions may be more difficult to aspirate.

Ancillary Studies

- Vimentin+, MSA(+), calponin(+)
- Cytokeratin(−), S100(−), and CD34(−), desmin(−), caldesmon(−).

Differential Diagnosis

- Sarcomas with myxoid changes,
- Myxoma,
- Neurofibroma, and schwannoma

Summary and Key Features

- Rapidly growing spindle cell lesion in adults with mixed cellular pattern (spindle, stellate fibroblast, polygonal, inflammatory) and mixed morphological pattern (myxoid, edematous, dense, hypo and hypercellular).

Myoselitis Ossificans with Myxoid Changes (Fig. 5.3)

- Myositis ossificans is a reparative pseudosarcomatous lesion that is distinguished by the presence of metaplastic bone formation.
- Occurs in a younger patient population than the other pseudosarcomas.
- Frequently affects healthy, active adolescents with history of trauma.
- Arises mainly in the subcutis and musculature of the upper and lower extremities.
- Rarely in unusual sites, including the mesentery and abdominal cavity.
- A painless, hard, well-demarcated mass averaging 3–6 cm.

Histology

- A well-delineated tan mass that has a soft, glistening center and a firm, gray, gritty periphery.
- Cellular spindle cell lesion consisting of tissue similar to that in nodular fasciitis, but with bone metaplasia in the periphery.
- Morphologic zonation becomes apparent:
  - The center retains its mixture of fibroblasts, abundant mucopolysaccharides (myxoid areas), and delicate collagen fibers

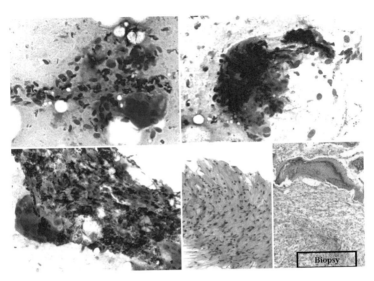

FIG. 5.3. Myositis ossificans with myxoid changes (DQ smears, *upper left & right* ×400, *lower left* ×200, Pap-stained smear, *lower middle* ×200, and section of excisional biopsy (H&E, *lower right* ×100). The smears show predominance of bland-appearing spindle cells with smooth nuclear membranes and evenly distributed chromatin, granular, fibrillar and myxoid background. Also seen are numerous plasmacytoid and polygonal osteoblasts and multinucleated osteoclasts. No osteoid or chondroid seen. Few fragmented muscle fibers seen and fragments of bone (*lower left*) also noted. The excisional biopsy confirmed the diagnosis (*lower right*) and showed zonations of the lesion with bony trabeculae present in the peripheral zone.

- Adjacent intermediate zone that contains osteoblasts, which form ill-defined trabeculae of woven bone.
- Peripheral zone, the bony trabeculae, undergoes remodeling and mineralization which resembles cancellous bone.
- Thin layer of loose fibrous tissue.

Cytomorphology

- High or low cellularity smears with spindle cells, fragments of muscle, osteoblasts, giant cells, and bone.

- The predominant cell type is spindle cells similar to nodular fasciitis.
- Granular, fibrillar and myxoid background.
- Plasmacytoid or polygonal osteoblasts and multinucleated osteoclasts.
- Osteoid or chondroid are absent.
- Bland nuclear features with smooth nuclear membranes and an even chromatin pattern.
- Fragmented muscle fibers.

Ancillary Studies: Same as Nodular Fasciitis

- Vimentin+, MSA(+), calponin(+)
- Cytokeratin(−), S100(−), and CD34(−), desmin(−), caldesmon(−).

Differential Diagnosis

- Osteosarcoma

Ganglion Cyst (Fig. 5.4)

- Most common location is the dorsal surface of the wrist.
- Young patients with female predominance.
- Unilocular or multilocular mass.
- May be associated with mild pain or functional impairment.
- The majority measures 1.5–2.5 cm.
- Adjacent to a joint capsule or tendon sheath.
- May arise from excessive mucin produced by fibroblasts.
- Does not communicate with joint spaces.

Histology

- A ganglion cyst usually presents as a superficial, firm, circum-scribed mass populated by benign-appearing histiocytes.
- Thick-walled cystic lesion surrounded by myxoid area.
- Myxoid area extends into surrounding soft tissue.

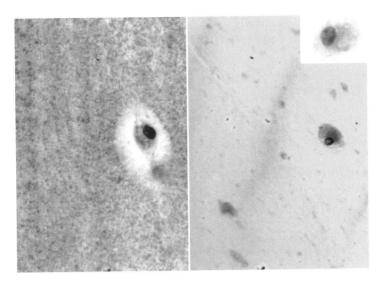

FIG. 5.4. Ganglion cyst (DQ smear, *left* ×200, Pap-stained smear, *right* ×200) presented as proximal mass of left hand from a 45-year-old male. The specimen was described as clear gel-like thick fluid. The smears are hypocellular and show viscous fluid that stain dark blue/magenta on Diff-Quik and light green on the Pap stain. The histiocytes are single and in small groups. They have frothy cytoplasm and round to bean-shaped nuclei. No cytological atypia seen. No capillary fragments seen. The specimen was signed out as hypocellular myxoid lesion, ganglion cyst vs. myxoma. The excisional biopsy of the lesion confirms a ganglion cyst.

Cytomorphology of Ganglion Cyst[3–5]

- A viscous fluid that stains dark blue/magenta on Diff-Quik and light green on the Pap stain.
- A paucicellular specimen with histiocytes residing in a prominent granular and mucinous background.
- The mucinous material may be seen as a folded pattern, mimicking crinkled plastic food wrap.
- The histiocytes are most often single, but small groups can also be seen.
- The histiocytes have frothy cytoplasm and round to bean-shaped nuclei.

- Occasional giant cells.
- No capillary fragments are seen.

Ancillary Studies

CD68+, CK−

Differential Diagnosis

- Myxoma
- Myxoid liposarcoma
- Myxoid malignant fibrous histiocytoma
- Extraskeletal myxoid chondrosarcoma (EMC)

Myxoma (Figs. 5.5 and 5.6)

- Benign soft tissue neoplasms present as slow-growing, painless, solitary masses in the skeletal muscle of the thigh.
- Can occur elsewhere and are usually subclassified by their location in the soft tissue into three types: intramuscular myxoma (IM), cutaneous myxoma (CM), and juxta-articular myxoma (JM).
- Multiple myxomas can be associated with familial conditions, such as McCune–Albright Syndrome, Carney's complex, and fibrous dysplasia.
- On imaging, myxomas can show an infiltrative border, which may lead to FNA biopsy, surgical biopsy, or excision. Excision is curative, since these are benign neoplasms and rarely recur.

Histology

- Mucoid, slimy gross appearance, within skeletal muscle
- Hypocellular with bland spindle cells (fibroblast-like)
- Aggregates of foamy histiocytes, a hypovascular lesion
- An abundant myxoid matrix

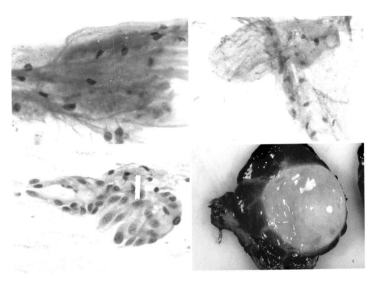

FIG. 5.5. Intramuscular Myxoma (DQ ×200 smear, *upper left*, Pap-stained smears, *right upper* ×100, and *left lower* ×200, and gross pathology of the excised lesion) presented as groin mass from a 55-year-old male. The specimen was described as clear gel-like thick fluid. The smears are hypocellular with spindle and polygonal/histiocytic cells in abundant myxoid background. The cells are isolated or in small clusters with spindle and columnar morphology associated with some foamy histiocytes. Some cells show long cytoplasmic processes with vacuolated cytoplasm. The subsequent excisional biopsy (*lower right*) shows intramuscular myxoma with relatively well-circumscribed borders with some peripheral infiltration and gelatinous mucoid homogenous cut surface.

- Bland spindle or stellate cells and rare muciphages within myxoid matrix
- Hypovascular lesion (scanty blood vessels) and no mitosis or necrosis
- Well-circumscribed with some peripheral infiltration between muscle
- Variants: cellular myxoma and juxta-articular myxoma (large joint)

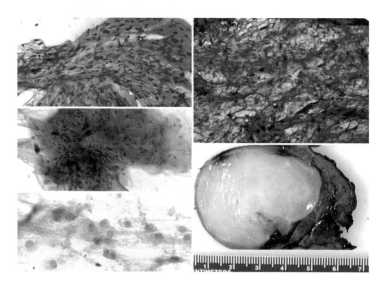

FIG. 5.6. Myxoma, cellular variant (DQ smear, *upper left* & *right* ×200, Pap-stained smears, *left middle* ×100 and *lower* ×200, and gross macroscopy of the excised lesion, *right lower*) presented as 5-cm posterior thigh mass from a 78-year-old female. The specimen was described as clear gel-like thick fluid. The smears are hypercellular with spindle and polygonal/histiocytic cells in abundant myxoid background. The cells are isolated or in small clusters with spindle and columnar morphology associated with some foamy histiocytes. Some cells show lipoblast-like morphology with vacuolated cytoplasm and indented nuclei. The specimen was signed out as myxoid tumor. The subsequent excisional biopsy (*lower right*) shows cellular variant of myxoma with relatively well-circumscribed borders and gelatinous mucoid homogenous cut surface.

Cytomorphology of Myxoma[3–7]

- Aspirate of droplets of clear glue-like fluid.
- Abundant myxoid background.
- Bland cells singly or in small clusters and foamy histiocytes.
- The cells may be round, polyhedral, triangular, long with cytoplasmic processes, with vacuolated cytoplasm.
- Atrophic muscle cells (multinucleated giant muscle cells) may be seen.

- Juxta-articular myxoma is a subtype and can demonstrate large size, hypercellularity, and infiltrative edges.
- Some cases of intramuscular myxomas may have areas of increased cellularity, increased collagen bundles, and more blood vessels (cellular myxomas).
- Soft tissue ganglia can also appear similar to soft tissue myxomas.

Ancillary Studies

Vimentin+, S100−, desmin−

Differential Diagnosis

- Nodular fasciitis
- Myxoid neurilemoma
- Ganglion
- Myxoid sarcomas (myxofibrosarcoma, fibromyxoid sarcoma, myxoid chondrosarcoma)

Neurilemoma/Schwannoma with Myxoid Features (Fig. 5.7)

- Majority of schwannomas arise in the head and neck.
- Can be found originating from nerves anywhere in the body.
- Usually is a well-circumscribed soft tissue lesion.
- Some cellular variants can appear as infiltrative and mimic sarcomas.

Histology

- A background of alternating hypocellular myxoid and cellular areas (Antoni A and B), and nuclear palisading in Verocay bodies.

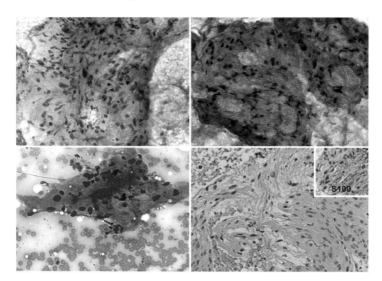

Fig. 5.7. Schwannoma/Neurilemoma with myxoid features (Pap-stained smears, *upper* ×200, DQ smear, *lower left* ×200, cell block H&E, *right lower* ×200, and S100 immunostain on cell block material, *inset, lower right*) presented as deltoid 2-cm mass from a 21-year-old-female. The smears are cellular with spindle cells in cohesive and delicate fibrillary and myxoid background. Numerous wavy, "fishhook" naked nuclei are seen. The smears, as well as the cell block, show two components: cellular component (Antoni A) that palisades (Verocay bodies), plus less cellular myxoid component (Antoni B). The immunostain of S100 is positive (*inset, lower right*).

- The nuclei are oval and comma-shaped.
- Strong and diffusely positive for S100, unlike the patchy weak positivity seen in malignant peripheral nerve sheath tumors (MPNST).
- "Ancient" and cellular variants of schwannoma may show variable atypia and pleomorphism, leading to possible false-positive diagnoses.
- The cytologic distinction between an ancient Schwannoma and well-differentiated MPNST can also be difficult. In general, MPNSTs usually have many mitotic figures and an absence of Verocay bodies, in addition to having anaplastic multinucleated cells, and only focal or patchy S100 positivity.

Cytomorphology of Neurilemoma/Schwannoma

- Cellular spindle cell smears in cohesive group.
- The spindle cell groups are flat, irregular, and of variable cellularity in an occasional myxoid-fibrillary matrix.
- The cellular smears show elongated ropy fascicles oriented in parallel and nuclear palisading.
- Two components: cellular component (Antoni A) that palisades (Verocay bodies), plus less cellular myxoid component (Antoni B).
- "Fishhook" naked nuclei, spindle cells, palisading
- Mast cells.
- Delicate fibrillary and myxoid background
- Occasional nuclear inclusions and mitotic figures

Ancillary Studies

Vimentin+, S100+, SMA−, desmin−

Differential Diagnosis

- Nodular fasciitis
- Myxoid neurofibroma
- Well-differentiated MPNST

Neurofibroma with Myxoid Features (Fig. 5.8)

- Neurofibromas and schwannoma are the most common benign neurogenic tumors.
- Neurofibromas most often occur in the superficial soft tissues.
- There is no predilection for any anatomic site.
- In the setting of neurofibromatosis, the tumors are multiple and often deep-seated.
- When arising from a large nerve, the neurofibroma is circumscribed but unencapsulated and is intertwined with the associated nerve trunk.

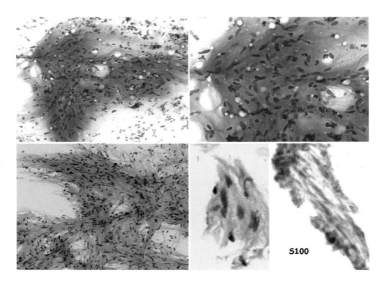

Fig. 5.8. Neurofibroma with Myxoid Features (DQ smears, *upper left* ×200 & *right* ×400, Pap-stained smears, *lower left* ×300, and cell block H&E ×400 and S100 immunostain, *right lower*) presented as 2-cm neck mass from 69-year-old female with history of cervical carcinoma and malignant melanoma. The smears are cellular and show cohesive groups sw of spindle cells with wavy nuclei and tapered end nuclei intermixed with collagen and myxoid background. No mitosis or necrosis. No distinct zonation, mainly spindle cells alternating with collagen and myxoid material. The specimen was signed out as benign neurogenic tumor, neurofibroma vs. schwannoma. The excisional biopsy shows 2-cm neurofibroma.

Histology

- Nonencapsulated; proliferation of all elements of peripheral nerves; Schwann cells with wire like collagen fibrils
- Wavy serpentine nuclei, pointed ends
- Stromal myxoid substances and mast cells
- Wagner–Meissner corpuscles, Pacinian corpuscles, axons, fibroblasts, and collagen; perineural cells of plexiform types; mitotic figures are rare
- May be infiltrative; less of a fascicular pattern than fibromatosis
- May have myxoid areas

- No Verocay bodies, no nuclear palisading, and no hyalinized thickening of vessel walls

Cytomorphology of Neurofibroma with Myxoid Features

- Spindle cell smears in cohesive group (less cellular than schwannoma).
- "Fishhook" wavy naked nuclei with tapered ends, while in schwannoma have rounded ends.
- Delicate fibrillary, collagenous and myxoid background.
- No significant mitoses, no necrosis.
- No distinct zonation and mainly spindle cells alternating with collagen and myxoid material.
- The spindle cells show features similar to those of schwannoma and similarly may show nuclear pleomorphism without mitotic activity.
- Rare neurofibroma may show presence of nuclear palisading.
- It may be difficult and unnecessary to distinguish schwannoma from neurofibroma on FNA diagnosis (can be signed out as benign neurogenic tumor, neurofibroma vs. schwannoma).

Ancillary Studies

Vimentin+, S100+, SMA−, Desmin−

Differential Diagnosis

- Nodular fasciitis
- Myxoid schwannoma
- Well-differentiated MPNST

Chondroma with Myxoid Features (Fig. 5.9)

- Chondromas are benign cartilage tumors developing within or on the surface of bones.
- They are composed of hyaline cartilage and located in the medullary cavity.

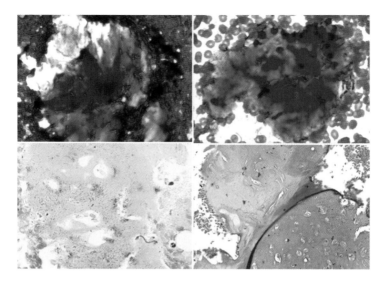

FIG. 5.9. Chondroma with myxoid changes, enchondroma (DQ smears, *upper* ×200, Pap-stained smears, *lower left* ×100, and cell block, H&E *right lower* ×100) presented as humerus mass from 43-year-old female. The smears show a fibrillary, magenta-purple cartilaginous and myxoid matrix containing bland nuclei with smooth contours and evenly dispersed chromatin. Some cells appear in lacunar spaces and have eccentric nuclei. Papanicolaou smears show dense and fibrillary fragments of green-blue cartilaginous and myxoid matrix. The cell block (*lower right*) shows moderate cellularity with uniform chondrocytes with small, round eccentric nuclei located within a purple-blue hyaline matrix. A rare binucleated chondrocyte is also present. The excisional biopsy was enchondroma with myxoid changes.

- 90% are solitary with ~60% located in the bones of the hand. Other frequent sites include tubular bones of feet, femur, tibia, humerus, fibula, and rib.
- Multiple lesions occur in the setting of Ollier's disease and Maffucci syndrome.
- Predominantly in adults, in third and fourth decades of life with equal gender distribution.
- Most are asymptomatic and found incidentally, though some may present with pain due to pathologic fracture.
- Arise superficially and present as a painless nodule.

- On imaging: arcs of calcification.
- They are usually treated with excision, with only rare reports of recurrences.

Histology

- They are composed of hyaline cartilage and located in the medullary cavity.
- Hypercellular cartilaginous nodules separated by collagenous bands.
- The chondrocytes can be binucleated or have enlarged nuclei.
- No/rare mitoses.
- Calcifications common and seen as a lace-like pattern.
- Myxoid material is rare and may show pleomorphic cells, worrisome for malignancy.
- The chondrocytes will stain positive for vimentin and S100.

Cytomorphology of Chondroma with Myxoid Features [4,5]

- Smears contain predominant cartilaginous matrix, often in large, sheet-like fragments or clumps, which appears strongly metachromatic on Romanowsky stain and may have a filmy, opaque or glassy appearance.
- Chondrocytes, located in the matrix within lacunar spaces, are round cells with a central, round, bland nucleus containing dense even chromatin and usually absent nucleoli. Cellular details may at times be obscured by cartilaginous matrix. A small quantity of single, bland chondrocytes may also be seen in the background.
- Within the lacunae, cells are usually single, though two closely opposed cells or rare double-nucleated chondrocytes may be seen. Multinucleated cells and mitotic figures are not seen.
- Multiple doublets, significant myxoid change, nuclear atypia, or necrosis suggest possibility of chondrosarcoma.

Ancillary Studies

- Vimentin+, S100+, SMA−, desmin−

Differential Diagnosis

- Chondrosarcoma, myxoid subtype
- Chondroid chordoma
- Myxoma

Myxoid Liposarcoma (Figs. 5.10a, b)

- Affect young adults

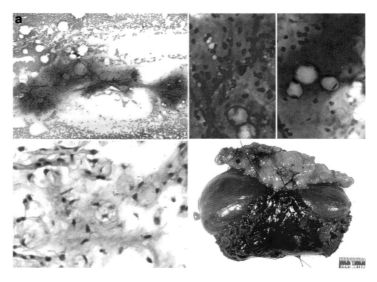

Fig. 5.10. (**a**) Myxoid liposarcoma (DQ smears, *upper left* × 100, *upper right* × 400, cell block, *lower left*, H&E × 300 and subsequent excisional biopsy (*right lower*) from a 30-year-old male who presented with a thigh mass that was thought by radiology to be myxoma. The aspirate yielded gel-like drops. The smears show an abundance of myxoid background and fragments of tissue with spindle or round vacuolated cells embedded in a myxoid matrix. Lipoblasts within tissue fragments with uni- or multivacuolated cytoplasm and indented nuclei are seen in smears (*upper right*) and cell block material (*lower left*). A branching network of capillary vessels was readily seen in smears as well as cell block material. No mitotic figures or necrosis. Ancillary studies, see next figure (Fig. 5.10b), confirmed liposarcoma. The excisional biopsy (*Lower right* showed myxoid liposarcoma.

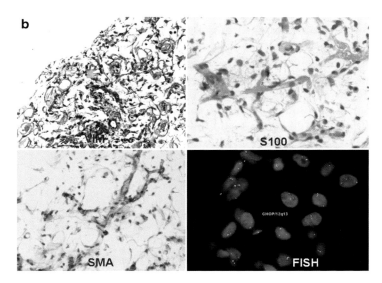

FIG. 5.10. (continued) (**b**) Ancillary studies on myxoid liposarcoma case of Fig. 5.10a performed on cell block material including vimentin (*upper left* × 200), S100 (*upper right* × 300) , SMA (*lower left* × 200), and FISH study on air-dried imprint cytology (*lower right*). The tumor cells are positive for vimentin, S100, and negative for SMA (only blood vessels were positive for SMA). The FISH study showed positivity for the CHOP genes, which is indicative of t(12;16)(q13;p11) reciprocal translocation causing the creation of a chimeric fusion protein CHOP-TLS. This study confirms the diagnosis of myxoid liposarcoma.

- Usually deep-seated well-circumscribed mass with a predilection for the thigh and popliteal fossa, and usually large
- Liposarcoma is the most frequent soft tissue sarcoma in adults
- Myxoid liposarcoma is a common variant of liposarcoma (33–50%)
- Rarely arises in the retroperitoneum
- Overall, approximately 30% of patients will develop metastases; however, the risk of metastases appears to be correlated with the cellularity of the lesion (greater cellularity implying greater risk of metastases). The metastatic lesions can occur in the lung, but also occur in extra-pulmonary locations as well (retroperitoneum, soft tissue, bone)

Histology

- Lipomatous tissue showing atypical cells with nuclear indentation caused by lipid-containing cytoplasmic vacuoles (lipoblasts).
- The characteristic feature of myxoid liposarcoma is the presence of thin-walled plexiform vessels coursing thru myxoid stroma with the neoplastic cells grouping close to the vessels ("chicken wire" or "crow's feet" pattern). This characteristic vasculature can be identified both in histologic sections and cytology smears.

Cytomorphology of Myxoid Liposarcoma

- Abundant myxoid background
- Fragments of tissue with spindle or round vacuolated cells embedded in myxoid matrix
- Lipoblasts within tissue fragment with uni- or multivacuolated cytoplasm and indented nuclei
- Rare single cells
- A branching network of capillary vessels
- No mitotic figures or necrosis

Ancillary Studies

- S100+, Vim+
- Both myxoid liposarcoma and round cell liposarcoma subtypes are related and share the unique t(12;16)(q13;p11) reciprocal translocation causing the creation of a chimeric fusion protein CHOP-TLS. About 10% of cases have the less common t(12;22) (q13;q12) translocation involving the CHOP and EWS genes

Differential Diagnosis

- Spindle cell lipoma with abundant myxoid matrix (no lipoblasts, not very vascular, spindle cells are CD34+, S100−)
- Intramuscular myxoma (no branching network of capillaries, no lipoblasts)

- Myxofibrosarcoma (nuclear atypia, thicker curvilinear capillaries)
- EMC (virtually avascular)

Myxofibrosarcoma/Myxoid MFH (Figs. 5.11 and 5.12)

- MFH is considered to be one of the most common soft tissue sarcomas in adults.
- Variety of histologic subtypes (pleomorphic, myxoid, giant cell, inflammatory).

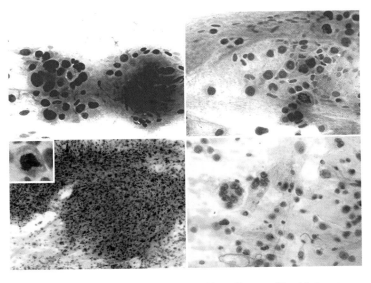

FIG. 5.11. Fibromyxoid sarcoma/myxoid malignant fibrohistiocytoma, MFH (DQ smears, *upper* × 400, Pap-stained smears, *lower left* × 200, *right* × 400) presented as 4-cm arm mass and lung mass from a 62-year-old female. The smears are abundantly cellular and demonstrate single and loosely cohesive clusters of highly atypical spindle and polygonal-round cells in an abundant mucinous background. The cells display pleomorphism and marked anisokaryosis. Nuclei have an irregular, coarse chromatin distribution. Admixed are large multinucleated giant cells and histiocyte-like cells having increased amounts of vacuolated cytoplasm. Also seen are a high number of mitotic figures including atypical mitoses (*lower, inset*). Few large pleomorphic cells are also seen. The subsequent histologic biopsy of both arm mass and lung mass confirm myxoid MFH.

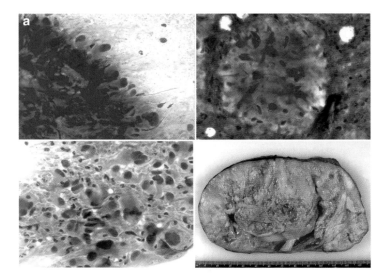

FIG. 5.12. (a) Fibromyxoid sarcoma/myxoid malignant fibrohistiocytoma, MFH, high-grade (DQ smears, *upper left* × 400, *right* × 300, Pap-stained smears, *lower left* × 400, and gross pathology of the excision, *lower right*) presented as 14-cm thigh mass from an 89-year-old female. The smears are abundantly cellular and demonstrate single and loosely cohesive clusters of highly atypical spindle, polygonal or round cells in an abundant mucinous background. The cells display marked pleomorphism and marked anisokaryosis. Nuclei have an irregular shape, with coarse chromatin distribution. Numerous large multinucleated giant cells and histiocyte-like cells are present. The subsequent excisional biopsy (*lower right*) showed high-grade myxoid MFH.

- Myxoid MFH is the second most common variant, after the pleomorphic subtype.
- It usually presents in older adults in the extremities or retroperitoneum, and is usually superficial with no gender predilection.
- Some lesions arise in the setting of orthopedic implants, Paget's disease, fibrous dysplasia, and bone infarcts.
- Associated with pathologic fracture in 25% of cases.
- Metaphyseal regions of long bones are the most frequently involved, as ill-defined lytic lesions with cortical expansion and breakthrough with minimal periosteal reaction.

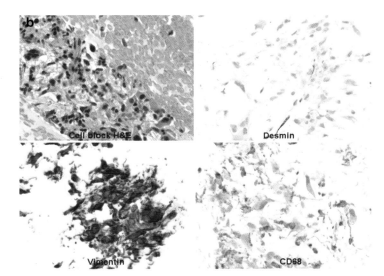

Fig. 5.12. (continued) (**b**) Cell block (*upper left*, H&E ×200) and immunostain study on cell block material of Desmin (*upper right*), vimentin (*lower left*), and CD68 (*lower right*) of the same case of Fig. 5.12a. The tumor cells are positive for vimentin and CD68 and negative for desmin.

- The superficial nature of this neoplasm can be a helpful distinguishing feature from the other myxoid soft tissue lesions that tend to be in deeper locations.
- MFH is a sarcoma that can metastasize to lymph nodes (the others are synovial sarcoma, clear cell sarcoma, rhabdosarcoma).
- These neoplasms are locally excised with wide margins.
- Better prognosis than pleomorphic MFH, over 50% recur, and about 25% metastasize.

Histology

- Grossly, variegated with hemorrhage and necrosis and permeative margins
- The combination of spindle-shaped, round, and giant cells are frequent cytologic features of MFH
- A nodular or lobulated architecture with prominent thick-walled curvilinear blood vessels
- At least 50% of the neoplasm should be myxoid

Cytomorphology of Myxoid MFH

- Abundant myxoid material with atypical vacuolated cells.
- The atypical cells may mimic lipoblasts.
- The atypical cells can vary from bland-appearing in the low-grade lesions to more pleomorphic in the high-grade lesions.
- Low-grade cases can mimic myxomas.
- Elongated fibroblast-like cells and histiocyte-like cells.

Differential Diagnosis

- Other myxoid tumors such as myxomas, myxoid fibrosarcomas, myxoid liposarcomas, myxoid leiomyosarcomas, myxoid chondrosarcoma, and chondromas
- Giant cell carcinoma from lung or pancreatic primary
- Benign fibrohistiocytic tumors: no malignant cells

Summary/Key Features

- Superficial tumor in adults with elongated fibroblast-like cells and histiocyte-like cells and giant cells with nuclear atypia in myxoid background

Extraskeletal Myxoid Chondrosarcoma: Fig. 5.13

- Primary chondrosarcomas comprise ~20% of malignant bone tumors and are the third most common primary bone malignancy after myeloma and osteosarcoma.
- There is a peak incidence in the fifth to seventh decades of life with a slight male predilection and the majority of patients being older than 50 years.
- Tumors typically present with local pain and/or swelling of long duration.
- Approximately 75% occur in the trunk and proximal portions of the femur and humerus with the most common skeletal sites being the pelvic bones (most frequently the ilium), proximal femur, proximal humerus, distal femur, and ribs.

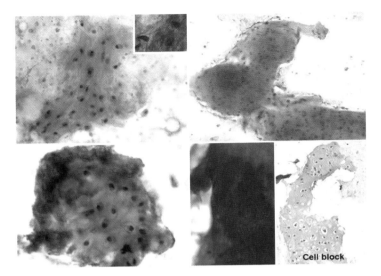

FIG. 5.13. Myxoid chondrosarcoma (DQ smears, *upper left* ×200, Pap-stained smears, *upper right* ×100 and *lower left* ×400, *middle* DQ ×200, and cell block H&E stain, *lower right* ×200) presented as lytic and focally calcified lesion in the left humerus from a 72-year-old male. The smears demonstrate fragments of a cellular myxoid matrix, which appeared magenta-purple on Romanowsky stain and greenish blue on Papanicolaou stain. The matrix appears focally watery and fibrillary in the myxoid area and more thick and dense areas with sharp borders in the chondroid matrix. The chondromyxoid matrix is hypercellular with mild to moderate cytologic atypia. The chondrocytes have distinct pink cytoplasm, central nuclei with evenly dispersed chromatin, and irregular nuclear contours with one to two small to indistinct nucleoli. The subsequent excisional biopsy confirmed myxoid chondrosarcoma.

- EMC are soft tissue neoplasms that predominantly occur in adulthood
- The most common location is in the deep soft tissues of the extremities
- It presents clinically as a painless or minimally tender, slow-growing mass
- High risk of local recurrence

Histology

- A lobulated myxoid tumor with nests or linear cords of small, round to oval cells
- A basophilic flocculent matrix lacking prominent vascularity
- There is no histologic grading of these neoplasms, since prognosis is largely dictated by clinical features

Cytomorphology of Extraskeletal Myxoid Chondrosarcoma[5–7]

- An abundance of extracellular matrix material is best appreciated on Romanowsky air-dried preparations, where it can appear watery with fibrillary/feathered edges to dense and thick with distinct borders. Hyaline cartilage fragments can also be seen.
- Cellularity and matrix composition depends on grade of neoplasm (higher grades usually correlate with increased cellularity and decreased matrix). Recognizable lacunae and binucleate forms can also be seen.
- A cord-like pattern in chondroid differentiation.
- Single chondrocytes can be widely scattered throughout the representative tissue or in clusters surrounding matrix material occasionally. Often a plasmacytoid configuration is identified with numerous, small cytoplasmic vacuoles.
- Nuclei are usually round to ovoid with slight degrees of hyperchromasia and enlargement (low-grade lesions). Cytoplasm is abundant and either finely granular or vacuolated. Higher grade tumors are enlarged with irregular nuclear contours, prominent nucleoli, and an open chromatin pattern.
- Chondrosarcoma can be difficult to differentiate from both chondroid and nonchondroid lesions: metastatic carcinoma (especially, renal cell carcinoma), chordoma, chondromyxoid fibroma, myxoma, and myxoid sarcoma.

Ancillary Studies

- S100+, EMA+, occasional NSE+, synaptophysin+
- Several chromosomal translocations that can be detected with FISH. The most common translocation is t(9;22)(q22;q12), which

involves the EWSR1 gene on chromosome 22q12. Thus, the EWSR1 (22q12) break-apart probe can be used for FISH testing in these tumors, but other neoplasms involving a translocation of chromosome 22 (Ewing sarcoma, t(11;22)(q24,q12); DSRCT, t(11;22) (p13;q12); clear cell sarcoma of soft parts, t(12,22)(q13;q12); and myxoid liposarcoma, t(12;22)) need to be ruled out.

Chordoma (Fig. 5.14a, b)[8-19]

- Arise from remnants of the notochord.
- Typically occur in the axial skeleton, sacrococcygeal region (50%), spheno-occipital region of the skull base (35%), and vertebral column (15%).

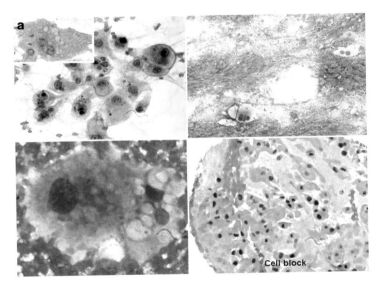

FIG. 5.14. (**a**) Chordoma (Pap-stained smear, *upper* ×400, DQ smears, *upper right* ×100 and *lower left* ×400, and cell block H&E stain, *lower right* ×300) presented as sacral mass from an 84-year-old female. The smears show abundant myxoid matrix which appear in thick gel-like globules. There are numerous numbers of physaliphorous cells (large vacuolated cells with atypical indented nuclei), and numerous mononuclear cells with granular cytoplasm. The physaliphorous cells have abundant, dense, purple, intracytoplasmic material (on DQ stain) and a magenta mucinous background.

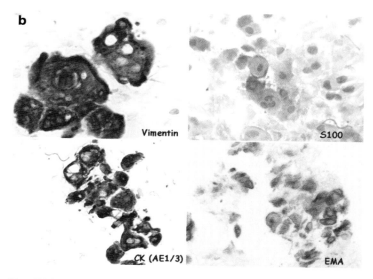

FIG. 5.14. (continued) (**b**) Chordoma immunostain study on cell block material of the case in Fig. 5.14a (vimentin, *upper left*, S100, *upper right*, cytokeratin, *lower left*, and EMA, *lower right*). Tumor cells stain positively for vimentin, S100, cytokeratin, and EMA. This immunoprofile confirms the diagnosis of chordoma.

- A subtype of chordoma, called the chondroid chordoma, most commonly occurs in the skull base. It usually arises in adulthood and presents with pain and neurologic defects.
- The chordomas in the sacrum have the best prognosis and overall survival. Metastases can occur, but tend to occur late in the clinical course.
- Classification: Conventional (most common), chondroid, and dedifferentiated/sarcomatous.

Histology

- It can be separated into conventional, chondroid, and dedifferentiated variants.
- The conventional type has a lobulated growth pattern that infiltrates the bone marrow and extends into soft tissue.

- The cells are large epithelioid cells in nests that may show cell-in-cell pattern and have eosinophilic cytoplasm.
- There are a variable number of cells, called physaliphorous cells, which have many vacuoles in the cytoplasm and appear "bubbly."

Cytomorphology of Chordoma[8]

- Abundant myxoid matrix which can appear string-like or in thick globules
- Variable numbers of physaliphorous cells
- Small mononuclear cells with granular cytoplasm
- On Diff Quick stains, the physaliphorous cells have abundant, dense, purple, intracytoplasmic material, and the background substance is usually magenta

Ancillary Studies

- S100+, EMA+, and CK+

Differential Diagnosis

- Myxoid chondrosarcoma (S100+, EMA+, CK−)
- Metastatic mucinous carcinoma (S100−, EMA+, CK+)

Low-grade Fibromyxoid Sarcoma(Fig. 5.15)[6,7,10,19]

- First reported by Evans in 1987 as unique tumors that were characterized by a deceptively bland histology and an indolent metastasizing course.
- Predominately occurs in younger patients (ages 26–46 years).
- Usually arises in the deep soft tissues of the thigh, inguinal region, shoulder, and perineum.
- Rare sites such as rib and others reported.
- Tends to recur and may also metastasize

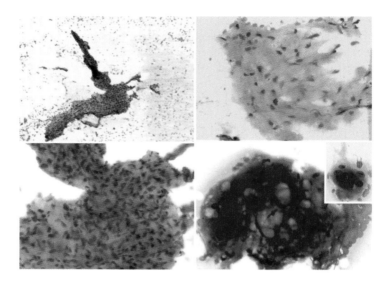

FIG. 5.15. Low-grade fibromyxoid sarcoma (Pap-stained smears, *upper left* × 100 *and lower left* ×300, *upper right* ×300, and DQ smear, *lower right* ×200) presented as a rib lesion from a 43-year-old female. The smears demonstrate fragments of a cellular myxoid matrix which appear magenta-purple on DQ stain and greenish blue on Papanicolaou stain. The cellularity is moderate. The capillary background is appreciated in the DQ smear (*lower right*). The spindle cells are relatively bland cytologically, with ovoid to tapered nuclei. Occasional giant cells are noted (*inset*). No dense stromal fragments present. This case was signed out as myxoid spindle cell tumor. The surgical excision confirmed low-grade fibromyxoid sarcoma.

- It should be distinguished from low-grade examples of myxofib-rosarcoma/myxoid MFH, which usually occurs in older patients, contains more pleomorphism, and seldom metastasizes

Histology

- Well circumscribed macroscopically
- Nonfascicular, whirled arrangement of fibroblastic-appearing cells within alternating areas of myxoid and fibrous stroma
- Low to moderate cellularity
- The neoplastic cells are bland fibroblastic cells with minimal nuclear pleomorphism

- Rare mitotic figures
- Rich capillary network in the myxoid areas within an otherwise hypovascular tumor
- Microscopic infiltration into the surrounding soft tissues

Cytomorphology of Low Grade Fibromyxoid Sarcoma

- A myxoid lesion with low cellularity
- The rich capillary background is not usually appreciated in the smears (rare capillary-type blood vessels)
- Spindle cells with relatively bland, ovoid to tapered nuclei consistent with a fibroblastic origin
- No dense stromal fragments (no fibrous component of this tumor)
- Majority of the cases signed out as myxoid spindle cell lesion/tumor

Ancillary Studies

- Vimentin+, SMA−, MSA−, Desmin−, S-100−, CD34−
- This neoplasm, like low-grade fibromyxoid sarcoma, has the identical characteristic translocation t(7;16)(q33;p11) with a fusion of the FUS gene to CREB3L2

Differential Diagnosis

- Fibromatosis (positive nuclear beta-catenin), and architecture with sweeping fascicles, rather than the swirling or vague storiform pattern of LGFS
- Other myxoid soft tissue lesions such as low-grade myxofibrosarcoma, myxoma, myxoid neurofibroma, and aggressive angiomyxoma

Metastatic Mucinous Carcinoma (Figs. 5.16a, b and 5.17)

- Mucinous carcinomas can arise from a variety of primary sites, including the stomach, colon, appendix, pancreas, ovary, breast, etc.
- Usually older patients

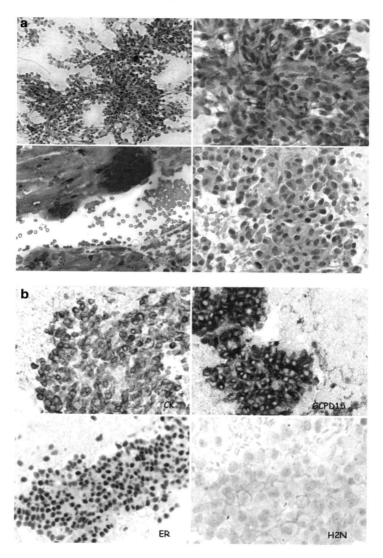

FIG. 5.16. (a) Metastatic mucinous carcinoma (Pap stained smear, *upper* ×100, *upper right* ×400, DQ, *lower left* ×200, and cell block H&E stain, *lower right* ×300) from a 75-year-old female, with no history of malignancy, presented with a pathological fracture of left humerus.

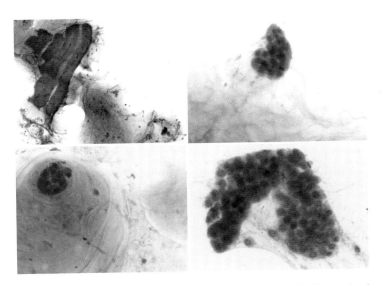

FIG. 5.17. Metastatic mucinous carcinoma of gastric origin (Pap-stained smear, *upper left* ×100, *upper right* ×300, *and lower right* ×400, and DQ, *lower left* ×300) from a 49-year-old female who presented with pelvic soft tissue mass. The smears are hypocellular, but with abundant extracellular mucin around floating neoplastic epithelial cells. The epithelial cells are cohesive, in small and large clusters. Few papillary-like fragments are also seen (*lower right*). The cells have moderate cytological atypia and moderate crowding of nuclei. Reviewing the pathology of the gastric tumor reveals mucinous adenocarcinoma with similar morphology.

Fig. 5.16. (continued) The smears are hypercellular with extracellular mucin present. The epithelial cells are loosely cohesive with plasmacytoid cells showing moderate nuclear atypia. Few osteoclast cells and osteoblasts are also present (*lower left*). The cell block shows atypical epithelial cells with grey mucoid material in the background. Immunostain study on cell block (see Fig. 5.16b) confirms metastasis from breast primary. (**b**) Ancillary study on mucinous carcinoma presented as pathological fracture of left humerus (case in Fig. 5.16a). The tumor cells stain positively for cytokeratin (*upper left*), GCPD15 (*upper right*), ER in >90% of tumor nuclei (*lower left*), and negatively for Her2Neu (+1, *lower right*). This immunoprofile confirms breast primary.

Histology

- Abundant mucinous material with epithelioid cells floating.
- The cells arranged singly or in small clusters.
- Signet-ring features may be seen.
- Can have dyscohesive cells.
- Variable nuclear atypia.
- Should be always in the differential of myxoid soft tissue lesions, and a positive cytokeratin immunostain can be helpful when performing a panel of immunohistochemical stains in these lesions.

Cytomorphology

- Abundant extracellular mucin around neoplastic epithelial cells.
- The epithelial cells can be dyscohesive, in small clusters, in papillary fragments, or in sheets.
- Signet-ring cell forms may be seen.
- Variable nuclear atypia.

Ancillary Studies

- CK+, EMA+, CEA+, Mucicarmine+
- Breast origin: ER+, PR+, Mama globulin+
- G.I.: CK20+, CK7−*, CEA+, CDx2+; (* stomach may express CK 7)
- Lung: CK7+, CK20−, TTF-1+ (in adenocarcinoma)

Differential Diagnosis

- Myxoid soft tissue lesions
- Myxoid soft tissue tumors

Pitfalls of Cytological Diagnosis of Myxoid Soft Tissue Lesions[19-22]

When cytologic aspirate smears contain an abundance of myxoid material, a variety of entities enter the differential diagnosis. The majority of neoplasms fall into the category of soft tissue neoplasms with myxoid features. However, there are also a variety of non-neoplastic changes that we have seen on aspirates of soft tissue lesions that may mimic myxoid soft tissue neoplasms. One of the most striking examples was myxoid degeneration of the soft tissue surrounding nonmyxoid neoplasia, which was suspicious for myxoid liposarcoma on immediate assessment (see Fig. 5.18),

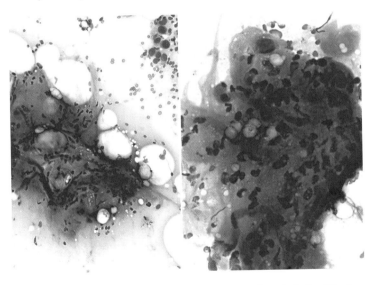

FIG. 5.18. Pitfalls of FNA of myxoid soft tissue lesions (misclassification of malignancy, DQ stained smears, *left* ×200, *right* ×400). The specimen was from a soft tissue mass from a patient with a high-grade lymphoma. This case was called myxoid liposarcoma on the initial assessment of the case due to the presence of myxoid adipose tissue with lipoblast-like cells and isolated highly atypical cells. The ancillary study failed to support that diagnosis and the final diagnosis was high-grade lymphoma associated with myxoid degeneration of surrounding adipose tissue.

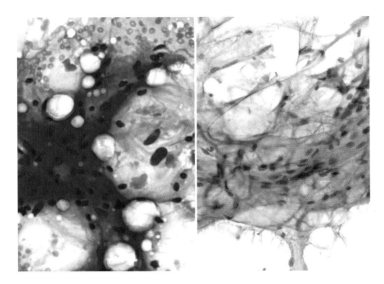

Fig. 5.19. Pitfalls of FNA of myxoid soft tissue lesions (false-positive myxoid liposarcoma, DQ, *left* ×200, and Pap-stained smear *right* ×200). Fibrolipoma with myxoid change was initially called myxoid liposarcoma (false-positive case). Numerous lipoblast-like cells are associated with capillary vessels and myxoid background. It is recommended that a positive diagnosis of myxoid liposarcoma should only be rendered with ancillary study results, particularly FISH, that can be performed easily on cytological material (air-dried smear or cell block sections).

and false-positive of myxoid liposarcoma from presence of myxoid changes and lipoblasts-like cells in the specimen (see Figs. 5.19 and 5.20). Another pitfall of myxoid changes is overcalling seroma as a myxoid lesion. Seroma is a collection of fluid in a previous cavity of surgical biopsy. The FNA of a seroma generally shows a clear yellow fluid that is paucicellular containing only a few degenerating foam cells. The background is edematous rather than mucinous. Squamous metaplasia of the cells lining in a seroma cavity appears to be a very rare event. The history is very essential for proper diagnosis (Fig. 5.21).

In summary, the diagnostic approach to these myxoid lesions involves clinical history, immunohistochemical stains, and molecular analysis, in conjunction with the cytomorphology, due to the cytomorphologic overlap in many of these entities.

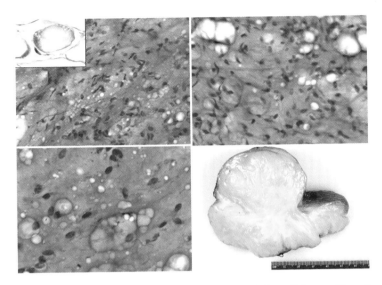

FIG. 5.20. Pitfalls of FNA of myxoid soft tissue lesions (false-positive of myxoid liposarcoma, DQ, *upper left* × 100, *upper right* × 200 *and lower left* × 400, and macroscopy of the excisional biopsy, *lower right*). A case of hibernoma that was called myxoid liposarcoma on FNA cytology due to the presence of pseudo lipoblasts and myxoid changes. It is recommended that positive diagnosis of myxoid liposarcoma should only be rendered if ancillary studies, particularly FISH study, are confirmatory. These studies can be performed easily on cytological material (air-dried smear or cell block sections).

Summary

Benign Differential and Key Features

Entity	Key Features
Nodular fasciitis	No atypical mitotic figures, rare single cells, short duration, rapid growth
Myxoma	Lack of vasculature, no atypia, hypocellular, muciphages
Schwannoma	Fishhook naked nuclei, spindle cells, Verocay bodies (palisading)
Neurofibroma	Fishhook naked nuclei, spindle cells, no Verocay bodies
Seroma	Surgical history, location at surgical cavity, edema, histiocytes
Ganglion Cyst	Location at hand near joint, hypocellular, myxoid background

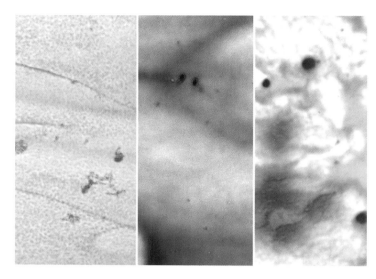

FIG. 5.21. Pitfalls of FNA of myxoid soft tissue lesions (false-positive of myxoid lesion, DQ, *left* ×100 *and middle* ×100, and Pap-stained smear, *right* ×200). This is a case of seroma in patient who had surgery in the neck for malignant melanoma. The lesion is cystic and it is in the previous biopsy site. The aspirated material was yellow fluid. Few histiocytes are present with no malignant cells seen. The background is edematous rather than mucinous/myxoid. In conjunction with clinical history, this case should be diagnosed as seroma and not a myxoid lesion.

Malignant Differential and Key Features

Entity	Key Features
Myxofibrosarcoma or myxoid MFH	Subcutis (not deep) thick-walled curvilinear blood vessels, large pleomorphic fibroblasts without indented nuclei
Myxoid liposarcoma	Thin-walled plexiform vasculature, lipoblasts with indented nuclei by fat vacuoles, no large bizarre cellular atypia; t(12;16) or t(12;22)
Extraskeletal myxoid chondrosarcoma (EMC)	Lack of vasculature, round monomorphic cells, cords/trabeculae of cells; t(9;22)
Low-grade fibromyxoid sarcoma	Bland spindle cells, tends to recur and metastasize, t(7;16)

(continued)

(continued)

Entity	Key Features
Chordoma	Myxoid matrix in thick globules, physaliphorous (bubbly) cells
Metastatic (mucinous) carcinomas	Cohesive clusters, atypical epithelioid cells floating in mucin

References

1. Rekhi B, Bhatnagar A, Bhatnagar D, et al. Cytomorphological study of soft tissue neoplasms: role of fluorescent immunocytochemistry in diagnosis. *Cytopathology*. 2005;16:219–226.
2. Downs-Kelly E, Goldblum JR, Patel RM, et al. The utility of fluorescence in situ hybridization (FISH) in the diagnosis of myxoid soft tissue neoplasms. *Am J Surg Pathol*. 2008;32(1):8–13.
3. Wakely PE, Bos GD, Mayerson J. The cytopathology of soft tissue myxomas: Ganglia, Juxta-articular myxoid lesions, and intramuscular myxoma. *Am J Clin Pathol*. 2005;123:858–865.
4. Thool AA, Raut WK, Lele VR, et al. Fine needle aspiration cytology of soft tissue chondroma: a case report. *Acta Cytol*. 2001;45:86-88.
5. Jakowski JD, Wakely PE. Cytopathology of extraskeletal myxoid chondrosarcoma: report of 8 cases. *Cancer Cytopathol*. 2007;111(5):298–305.
6. Silverman J, Nathan G, Olson PR, et al. Fine-needle aspiration cytology of low-grade fibromyxoid sarcoma of the renal capsule (capsuloma). *Diagn Cytopathol*. 2000;23(4):279–283.
7. Vernon SE, Bejarano PA. Low-grade fibromyxoid sarcoma: a brief review. *Arch Pathol Lab Med*. 2006;130:1358–1360.
8. Lefer LG, Rosier RP. The cytology of chordoma. *Acta Cytol*. 1978;22(1):51–53.
9. Fletcher CDM, Unni KK, Mertens F. *Pathology and Genetics of Tumors of Soft Tissue and Bone*. France: IARC Press; 2002:237–239.
10. Lindberg GM, Maitra A, Gokaslan ST, et al. Low grade fibromyxoid sarcoma: fine-needle aspiration cytology with histologic, cytogenetic, immunohistochemical, and ultrastructural correlation. *Cancer*. 1999;87(2):75–82.
11. Bergh P, Kindblom LG, Gunterberg B, et al. Prognostic factors in chordoma of the sacrum and mobile spine: a study of 39 patients. *Cancer*. 2000;88(9):2122–2134.
12. Boriani S, Bandiera S, Biagini R. Chordoma of the mobile spine: fifty years of experience. *Spine*. 2006;31(4):493–503.

13. Brandal P, Bjerkehagen B, Danielsen H. Chromosome 7 abnormalities are common in chordomas. *Cancer Genet Cytogenet*. 2005;160(1):15–21.

14. Breteau N, Demasure M, Lescrainier J, et al. Sacrococcygeal chordomas: potential role of high LET therapy. *Recent Results Cancer Res*. 1998;150:148–155.

15. Casali PG, Messina A, Stacchiotti S. Imatinib mesylate in chordoma. *Cancer*. 2004;101(9):2086–2097.

16. Cheng EY, Ozerdemoglu RA, Transfeldt EE, et al. Lumbosacral chordoma. Prognostic factors and treatment. *Spine*. 1999;24(16):1639–1645.

17. Chugh R, Tawbi H, Lucas DR, et al. Chordoma: the nonsarcoma primary bone tumor. *Oncologist*. 2007;12:1344–1350.

18. York JE, Kaczaraj A, Abi-Said D, et al. Sacral chordoma: 40-year experience at a major cancer center. *Neurosurgery*. 1999;44(1):74–79. discussion 79–80.

19. Akerman Mans, Domanski Henryk. *The Cytology of Soft Tissue Tumors*, vol. 16. Switzerland: Karger; 2003:83–84.

20. Silverberg Steven, DeLellis Ronald, Frable William, LiVolsi Virginia, Wick Mark. *Silverberg's Principles and Practice of Surgical Pathology and Cytopathology*, vol. 1. 4th ed. China: Elsevier Inc; 2006:388.

21. Klijanienko J, Caillaud JM, Lagacé R. Comparative fine-needle aspiration and pathologic study of malignant fibrous histiocytoma: cytodiagnostic features of 95 tumors in 71 patients. *Diagn Cytopathol*. 2003;29(6):320–326.

22. Klijanienko J, Caillaud J, Lagacé R. Fine-needle aspiration of primary and recurrent benign fibrous histiocytoma: classic, aneurysmal, and myxoid variants. *Diagn Cytopathol*. 2004;31(6):387–391.

6

Cytopathology of Soft Tissue Lesions with Predominance of Epithelioid, Round/Polygonal Cells, Glandular Cells, Inflammatory Cells

Živa Pohar-Marinšek[1] and Walid E. Khalbuss[2]
[1]Department of Cytopathology, Institute of Oncology, Ljubljana, Slovenia, EU
[2]University of Pittsburgh Medical Center, UPMC-Shadyside, POB2, Suite 201 Cytology, 5150 Centre Avenue, Pittsburgh, PA 15232, USA

This group of lesions includes benign and malignant tumors as well as some nontumorous conditions. Some lesions are composed predominantly or entirely of one morphological cell type while others contain two or more types. The majority of these lesions are composed primarily of soft tissue while some are metastases or direct extensions from processes in the surrounding skin, visceral organs, or bones.

Soft tissue lesions with predominance of epithelioid cells:

- Rhabdomyoma
- Granular cell tumor
- Epithelioid sarcoma
- Epithelioid variants of leiomyosarcoma
- Malignant peripheral nerve sheath tumor
- Angiosarcoma
- Epithelioid hemangioendothelioma

W.E. Khalbuss and A.V. Parwani, *Cytopathology of Soft Tissue and Bone Lesions*, Essentials in Cytopathology 9, DOI 10.1007/978-1-4419-6499-1_6, © Springer Science+Business Media, LLC 2011

- Malignant extrarenal rhabdoid tumor (ERT)
- Pleomorphic rhabdomyosarcoma (PR)
- Clear cell sarcoma
- Alveolar soft part sarcoma
- Metastatic tumors (melanoma, carcinoma, mesothelioma)
- Some types of lymphomas

Soft tissue lesions with predominance of round cells:

- Rhabdomyosarcoma
- Ewing/PNET
- Neuroblastoma
- Desmoplastic small round cell tumor
- Poorly differentiated synovial sarcoma
- Cellular variant of extraskeletal myxoid chondrosarcoma (EMC)
- Paraganglioma
- Glomus tumor
- Solitary fibrous tumor
- Non-Hodgkin lymphoma.

Soft tissue lesions with predominance of inflammatory/reactive cells

- Abscess/granulomatous inflammation
- Proliferative fasciitis/myositis
- Focal myositis
- Fat necrosis
- Muscle regeneration.

Tumors with Predominance of Epithelioid/ Polygonal Cells

Rhabdomyoma (Adult Type) (Fig. 6.1)

A rare, benign tumor of muscle differentiation

- Predominantly within the head and neck region.
- Patients' ages range from 30 to 80 years with a male predominance.[1,2]
- Rhabdomyoma grows slowly and eventually causes dysphagia, hoarseness, and dyspnea due to obstruction of food and airway passages.
- There may be recurrence after local excision.

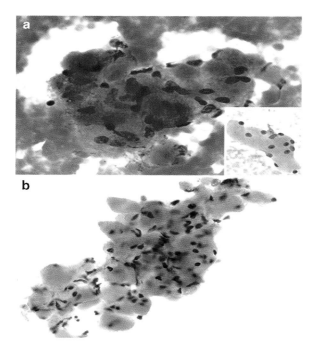

Fig. 6.1. *Adult rhabdomyoma*: Tumor cell groups showing large cells with abundant, granular cytoplasm. Nuclei are round or oval, uniform. Giemsa stain, ×400 (**a**). Papanicolaou stain, ×400 (**b**). The cell borders are indistinct giving cell groups a syncytial appearance. Nuclei contain prominent nucleoli (*inset*). Rhabdomyoma is a rare, benign tumor of muscle differentiation occurs predominantly within the head and neck region with a male predominance. It grows slowly and eventually causes dysphagia, and obstruction of food and airway passages. It is usually positive for desmin, alpha SMA, and myoglobin.

Cytomorphology of Adult Rhabdomyoma

- Smears are poorly to moderately cellular, composed of small cell groups and few dissociated cells in a clean or hemorrhagic background.[2–4]
- Tumor cells are large, round, and polygonal with abundant granular cytoplasm. Cell borders are usually distinct. Some small vacuoles may be seen. Cross-striations are present in rare cases.
- Nuclei are small, round with slight variation in size, located centrally or peripherally. Some cells appear multinucleated when

cellular borders are indistinct. Size of nucleoli varies from small to prominent.

Ancillary Studies

- Immunohistochemistry: positivity for desmin, alpha SMA, and myoglobin.

Differential Diagnosis

- Granular cell tumor and
- Hibernoma
- Normal striated muscle may also be confused with rhabdomyoma.[5] Immunocytochemistry is often necessary for a correct diagnosis.

Granular Cell Tumor (Fig. 6.2)

- A tumor of neuroectodermal origin located most commonly in the subcutaneous tissues and skin of middle age patients.
- It occurs at a wide variety of sites; however, tongue is the commonest location.
- Imaging data of granular cell tumors in breast suggest carcinoma.[6]
- The majority of granular cell tumors are benign and do not recur if excised properly.
- Rare malignant granular cell tumors also exist but there are no definite histological or cytological criteria for separating them from their benign counterparts.[7]

Cytomorphology of Granular Cell Tumor: Benign

- Smears are usually moderately or highly cellular, composed mainly of dissociated cells and naked nuclei with few interspersed cell groups.[8]
- Cell groups have a syncytial appearance due to indistinct cytoplasmic borders.
- Some smears contain mainly naked nuclei and few preserved cells in a basophilic background derived from degenerated cytoplasm.
- Tumor cells are large, polygonal, oval, or round, with abundant, granular cytoplasm, and indistinct borders.[9]
- Nuclei can be small, round, and uniform, located centrally or peripherally. An alternative picture features mild to moderate anisonucleosis, hyperchromasia, and nucleoli.[6]

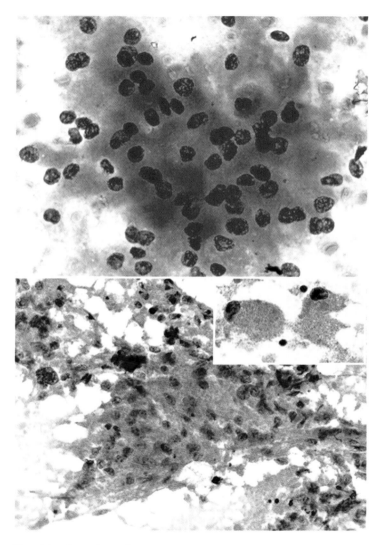

FIG. 6.2. *Granular cell tumor: benign.* Group of poorly preserved individual cells with syncytial appearance and indistinct cytoplasmic borders. Nuclei are round with coarse chromatin and nucleoli, Giemsa, ×600; Papanicolaou, ×400. Granular cell tumor is of neuroectodermal origin located in the subcutaneous tissues and skin of middle age patients with the tongue as the commonest location. It is usually positive for S-100 protein. Differential diagnosis includes adult rhabdomyoma and hibernoma.

Ancillary Studies

- Immunohistochemistry: positivity for S-100 protein.

Differential Diagnosis

- Differential diagnosis includes adult rhabdomyoma and
- Hibernoma.
- Tumors located in subcutaneous breast tissue may be mistaken for breast carcinoma when granular cells are poorly preserved or when they show nuclear atypia.

Cytomorphology of Granular Cell Tumor: Malignant (Fig. 6.3)

- Some malignant granular cell tumors are completely bland and indistinguishable from the benign ones.
- Certain reports state that hyperchromasia, increased nuclear/cytoplasmic ratio, nuclear pleomorphism, and spindle cell morphology are associated with malignancy when they are present diffusely.[10]
- The degree of atypia may not be more pronounced in malignant granular cell tumors as compared to atypia in benign granular cell tumors.

Epithelioid Sarcoma (Fig. 6.4)

- A malignant soft tissue tumor of unknown lineage affecting predominantly young adults with a predilection for males.
- The "distal" type is located mainly on the extremities while the "proximal" type is found in the pelvis, perineum, and genital area and behaves more aggressively.
- Clinical features are not remarkable; however, recurrence rate is high, and metastases appear in lungs and lymph nodes. Overall survival is poor.
- In histology the distal type is composed of a mixture of epithelioid and spindle cells with frequent areas of necrosis which imparts a pseudo granulomatous appearance and simulate a benign lesion. In the proximal type, epithelioid cells predominate and simulate carcinoma or ERT.

Cytomorphology of Epithelioid Sarcoma

- According to our experience, classical epithelioid sarcoma can rarely be mistaken for a benign lesion in cytology as it sometimes

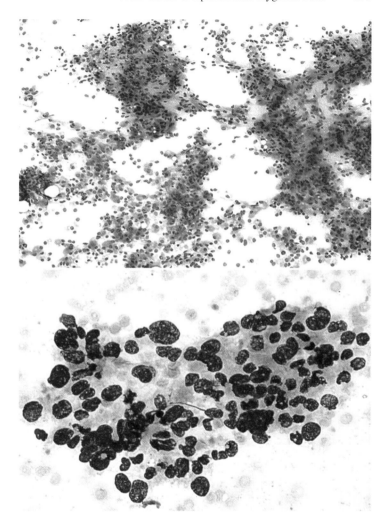

FIG. 6.3. *Malignant granular cell tumor*: A very cellular smear with tumor cells showing coarse chromatin, anisonucleosis, and scant cytoplasm. Giemsa stain ×100 and ×400, respectively. The degree of atypia may not be more pronounced in malignant granular cell tumors as compared to atypia in benign granular cell tumors.

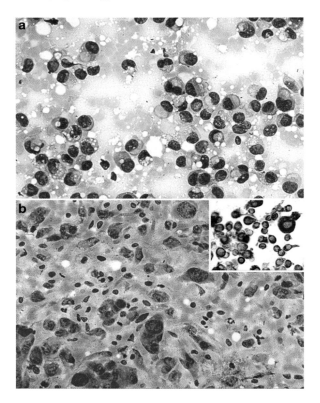

FIG. 6.4. *Epithelioid sarcoma*: (**a**) Dissociated tumor cells have a plasmacytoid appearance, some cells are binucleated. There is a pale perinuclear area due to whorls of intermediate filaments simulating secretory vacuoles of Adenocarcinoma. Giemsa stain ×400. (**b**) A polymorphic population of round, plasmacytoid and spindle cells with obvious anisonucleosis and hyperchromasia. There are some lymphocytes in the background. Giemsa stain, ×600. Positive immunocytochemical staining for cytokeratin (*inset*). It affects predominantly young adults with a predilection for males. The "distal" type is located mainly on the extremities while the "proximal" type is found in the pelvis, perineum, and in genital area and behaves more aggressively. Clinical features are not remarkable; however, recurrence rate is high, metastases appear in lungs and lymph nodes. Overall survival is poor.

happens in histology.[11] Even when many granulocytes are present, the malignant nature of the lesion is obvious.[12] However, some cytopathologists notice that epithelioid sarcoma can simulate an inflammatory process in scanty smears.[13]

- Cells are moderately large, round, or polygonal, well demarcated with abundant cytoplasm and eccentric nuclei. Some cells have cytoplasmic tails.
- There is a perinuclear pale zone in the cytoplasm of many cells, corresponding to whorls of filaments. Such cells, called rhabdoid, are more numerous in the proximal type of epithelioid sarcoma.[14]
- Nuclei are hypochromatic with coarse chromatin, round with smooth contour.
- The degree of anisonucleosis varies from uniform to moderately pleomorphic in different cases.[15]
- The number and size of nucleoli is also variable.
- There are a few binucleated and multinucleated cells.
- Inflammatory cells are usually not a prominent feature.
- Spindle cells are few in cases with abundant epithelioid cells.
- The rare fibroma-like variant, which is predominantly a spindle cell lesion, can look benign. Dissociated cells predominate; cell groups are few with no organoid structure. Some smears contain tissue fragments composed of stroma and tumor cells.[11]

Ancillary Studies

- Immunohistochemistry: positivity for keratin and EMA.

Differential Diagnosis

- Metastatic carcinoma,
- Melanoma, nodular hidradenoma of skin,
- Epithelioid leiomyosarcoma, epithelioid malignant peripheral nerve sheath tumor (MPNST).

Epithelioid Leiomyosarcoma (Fig. 6.5)

- Epithelioid morphology is very uncommon in leiomyosarcomas and is usually present in only part of the tumor. However, such areas can be relatively large and a cytological sample can consist solely of epithelioid cells. Epithelial morphology can predominate in metastatic lesions which are target of FNAC.[16]

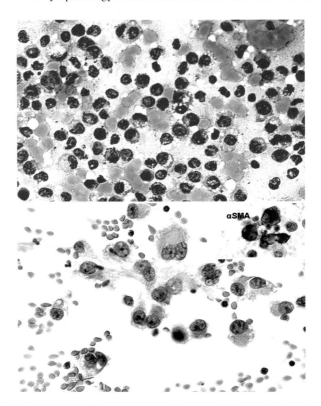

FIG. 6.5. *Epithelioid liemyosarcomas*: Tumor cells lie predominantly in a dissociated pattern with few tissue fragments. There is a mixture of oval and polygonal cells; however, some reports mention also spindle-shaped cells.[19] Anisonucleosis varies from slight to moderate. Hyperchromatic nuclei with coarse chromatin are positioned mainly at the periphery of cells and some cells are binucleated. Multinucleated cells are rare. Nucleoli are better appreciated in Papanicolaou staining; in some cases they are prominent.

- Epithelioid leiomyosarcomas can be found in the stomach wall, omentum, mesentery, retroperitoneum, and in skin and superficial subcutaneous tissues of various locations.[17,18]

Cytomorphology of Epithelioid Leiomyosarcoma

- Tumor cells lie predominantly in a dissociated pattern with few tissue fragments.

- There is a mixture of oval and polygonal cells; however, some reports mention also spindle-shaped cells.[19] Anisonucleosis varies from slight to moderate.
- Tissue fragments may contain abundant stroma, which stains pink in Giemsa.
- Cytoplasm is abundant and well demarcated.
- In some cells there is a lighter perinuclear area and small vacuoles are often noticed.
- Hyperchromatic nuclei with coarse chromatin are positioned mainly at the periphery of cells and some cells are binucleated. Multinucleated cells are rare. Nucleoli are better appreciated in Papanicolaou staining; in some cases they are prominent.[20]

Ancillary Studies

- Immunohistochemistry: positively for alpha SMA and desmin, keratin and EMA in majority of cases.
- Since positivity for epithelial antigens is usually focal the reactions can be negative in cytological samples.

Differential Diagnosis

- Epithelioid sarcoma and
- All epithelioid variants of other sarcomas Melanoma and
- Metastatic adenocarcinoma,
- Gastrointestinal stromal tumor.

Epithelioid Malignant Peripheral Nerve Sheath Tumor (Fig. 6.6)

This is a rare variant of MPNST which is not associated with fibromatosis.

- Epithelioid MPNST can be located in deep soft tissues or superficially in which case the prognosis is better.
- It can be composed entirely or partly of epithelioid cells.

Cytomorphology of Epithelioid MPNST

- Smears are moderately or highly cellular and composed of dissociated cells and cell groups. The overall picture can be monomorphous; some cases show moderate anisonucleosis.

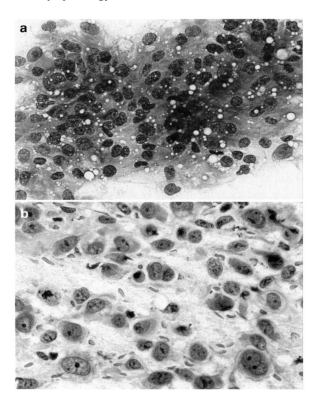

Fig. 6.6. *Epithelioid malignant peripheral nerve sheath tumor (MPNST)*: (**a**) Cellular smears with single cells and cell groups showing moderate anisonucleosis. Tumor cells are large, round or oval, with abundant cytoplasm while nuclei are usually positioned eccentrically. (**b**) Nuclei are hyperchromatic with coarse chromatin and can contain nucleoli. Cytoplasm is well delineated in preserved specimens. When cells are partly degenerated, cytoplasm blends into the background or is lost and naked nuclei prevail.

- Tumor cells are large, round or oval, with abundant cytoplasm while nuclei are usually positioned eccentrically.[21]
- Nuclei are hyperchromatic with coarse chromatin and may contain nucleoli.[22]
- Cytoplasm is well delineated in preserved specimens. When cells are partly degenerated, cytoplasm blends into the background or is lost and naked nuclei prevail.

- Cell groups are not numerous and have no organoid structure but nevertheless may simulate carcinoma.
- Spindle-to-ovoid cells have been reported in cell groups.[23]
- In some cases there is myxoid substance in the background between dissociated cells and within the cell groups.

Ancillary Studies

- Immunocytochemical reaction for keratin, EMA, and S-100 protein may be positive. The number of positive cells is variable and negative reaction is not unusual.

Differential Diagnosis

- Melanoma,
- Carcinoma,
- Epithelioid variants of other sarcomas,
- Synovial sarcoma if oval and spindle cells are also present.

Epithelioid Angiosarcoma (Fig. 6.7)

- Epithelioid angiosarcoma is a morphological variant of angiosarcoma which is seen more commonly in soft tissues and internal organs than in skin which is generally the most common location for angiosarcoma.[24]
- It is a malignant, high-grade tumor of adults, mostly elderly patients.
- Due to large hemorrhagic areas it can be radiologically mistaken for a hematoma. Poor yield in FNA samples described in cytological literature is also the result of degeneration and hemorrhage within the tumor.

Cytomorphology of Epithelioid Angiosarcoma

- Smears with adequate yield are composed predominantly of dissociated cells and variable number of cell groups.
- Groups can be loosely arranged or form rosettes or even papillae. These are called vasoformative structures and are believed to be

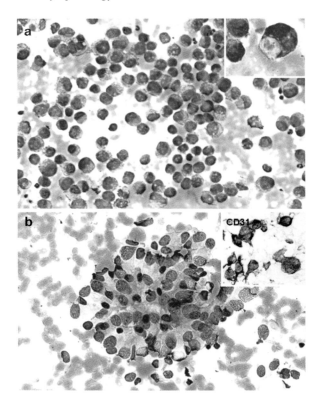

FIG. 6.7. *Epithelioid angiosarcoma*: (**a**) Smears compose dissociated cells and cell groups. Groups can be loosely arranged or may have a form of rosettes or even papillae (vasoformative structures). (**b**) Cells are large with abundant, well-delineated cytoplasm and hyperchromatic nuclei, many of them eccentrically positioned. Intracytoplasmic lumina are seen only in occasional cells. Cytoplasm can also contain small vacuoles and hemosiderin deposits. The background is usually very hemorrhagic. In ideal cases CD31 (insert) and CD34 are positive as well as epithelial markers (keratin and EMA).

pathognomonic by some authors.[25] In our opinion, they are indistinguishable from similar arrangements in adenocarcinomas.

- In general, cells are large with abundant, well-delineated cytoplasm and hyperchromatic nuclei, many of them eccentrically positioned.

- Anisocytosis varies from case to case. Some samples are very monomorphous with round nuclei and therefore reminiscent of a benign epithelial tumor.
- At the other end of the spectrum are pleomorphic epithelioid angiosarcomas showing prominent anisonucleosis with many bi and multinucleated cells, multiple nucleoli, and frequent mitoses. Such cases simulate poorly differentiated carcinomas.
- Nuclear contour also varies greatly from smooth[26] to irregular with prominent indentations.[27]
- Intracytoplasmic lumina are seen in occasional cells.[28] Some consider them pathognomonic; however, they resemble secretory vacuoles and may be misleading. Cytoplasm may also contain small vacuoles and hemosiderin deposits.
- The background is usually very hemorrhagic.

Ancillary Studies

- In ideal cases CD31 and CD34 are positive as well as epithelial markers (keratin and EMA). However, many cases may show only one of these markers.

Differential Diagnosis

- Other epithelioid sarcomas melanoma
- Adenomas,
- Carcinomas.
- In case there is secondary inflammation, tumor cells may be confused with histiocytes.[28]

Epithelioid Hemangioendothelioma (Fig. 6.8)

- Epithelioid hemangioendothelioma (EH) is a rare vascular tumor with an intermediate malignant potential.
- It arises from a vein, sometimes from an artery in superficial or deep-seated soft tissues mostly in the extremities in all age groups except in young children.
- EH are also found in internal organs such as lung and liver as well as in bones. Head and neck area is seldom affected with few cases reported in oral cavity.[29]
- Clinical symptoms include a painful tumor, sometimes associated with signs of edema and thrombophlebitis.

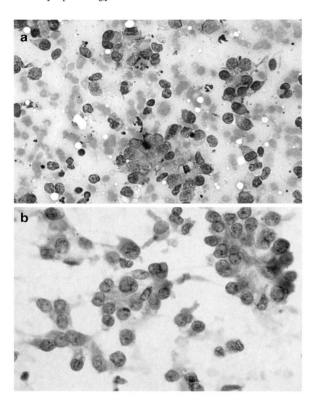

Fig. 6.8. *Epithelioid hemangioendothelioma*: (**a**) Cellular smears with predominance of single cells. The cells have abundant cytoplasm, and contain many small vacuoles or rarely larger vacuoles. Nuclei are round, some irregularly shaped and even lobular. There are binucleated and occasional multinucleated cells as well as mitotic figures. Small, multiple nucleoli are present. (**b**) Some cell groups have a glandular, rosette-like appearance or the shape of small sheets.

- Biological potential cannot be definitely predicted on the basis of morphology since EH without atypia have a metastatic potential of 17%.[30]

Cytomorphology of Epithelioid Hemangioendothelioma

- Cellularity of smears varies from scant to highly cellular. Dissociated cells predominate over cell groups.

- Cells are epithelioid with moderate variation in size. Cytoplasm is abundant and contains many small vacuoles in some cells and a larger vacuole in occasional cells.[29]
- Nuclei are predominantly round, some irregularly shaped and even lobular. There are binucleated and occasional multinucleated cells as well as mitotic figures.
- Small, multiple nucleoli are present.[31]
- Some cell groups have a glandular, rosette-like appearance[32] or occur in small sheets.
- Some smears contain fragments of metachromatic stroma in the background.[33]
- In our opinion EH cannot be distinguished cytologically from epithelioid angiosarcoma; however, some believe that morphologic features are distinctive.[34]

Ancillary Studies

- Immunohistochemistry: positivity for CD31, CD34, and factor VIII.

Differential Diagnosis

- Angiosarcoma,
- Melanoma,
- Metastatic carcinoma,
- Other epithelioid variants of various sarcomas.

Extrarenal Rhabdoid Tumor (Fig. 6.9)

- ERT is a rare malignant childhood neoplasm occurring in soft tissues of the neck and paraspinal locations as well as in liver and gastrointestinal tract. Some cases are congenital.[35]
- It is a highly aggressive neoplasm with dismal prognosis.

Cytomorphology of Extrarenal Rhabdoid Tumor

- Smears are usually very cellular, containing many dissociated cells and variable number of cell groups.
- Cells are medium sized and large, polygonal, plasmacytoid (rhabdoid) with abundant, well-demarcated cytoplasm.
- There are hyaline globules[36] in many cells and sometimes a lighter area which can resemble a secretory vacuole. In some smears, cytoplasm contains many small degenerative vacuoles.[37]

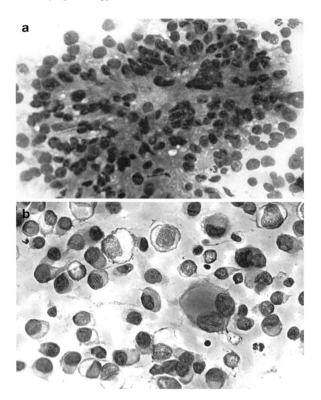

FIG. 6.9. *Extrarenal rhabdoid tumor:* (**a**) Highly cellular smears containing many dissociated cells and some cell groups. (**b**) Cells are medium sized and large, polygonal, plasmacytoid (rhabdoid) with abundant, well-demarcated cytoplasm. There are hyaline globules in many cells and sometimes a lighter area which can resemble a secretory vacuole. In some smears, cytoplasm contains many small degenerative vacuoles. Nuclei are round or somewhat irregular, hyperchromatic with prominent nucleoli. There is slight anisonucleosis, some binucleated, and occasional multinucleated cells. Cell groups have the form of sheets, clusters, or even rudimentary gland-like structures.

- Nuclei are round or somewhat irregular, hyperchromatic with prominent nucleoli. There is slight anisonucleosis, some binucleated, and occasional multinucleated cells.
- Cell groups have the form of sheets, clusters, or even rudimentary gland-like structures.

Ancillary Studies

- Immunohistochemistry: coexpression of epithelial antigens keratin and EMA, vimentin and occasionally also neuroectodermal antigens NSE, synaptophysin, and CD99.
- Alpha SMA has also been reported in ERT.

Pleomorphic Rhabdomyosarcoma (Fig. 6.10)

- PR is a malignant tumor of adults, most commonly during the sixth decade of life. Deep soft tissues of the lower extremities are most frequently affected; however, several other locations have been reported.
- Imaging shows the same consistency as skeletal muscles; necrotic areas can be identified.
- The prognosis is poor; there are no known prognostic factors.
- Histological patterns vary greatly and can be subdivided into classical, round cell, and spindle.[38]

Cytomorphology of Pleomorphic Rhabdomyosarcoma

- As in histology, morphological patterns vary also in cytology and some cases are composed of cells with predominantly rhabdoid features.
- Dissociated cells are numerous among few tissue fragments.
- Cells are large, round, oval, or polygonal with obvious variation in size. There are many binucleated cells and some multinucleated ones.
- Nuclei are hyperchromatic, eccentric, round with coarse chromatin, many irregularities of nuclear membrane and sometimes with prominent nucleoli.
- Cytoplasm is abundant, well delineated and contains a globular structure in many cells.
- Cross-striations have been reported in individual cases.[39]

Ancillary Studies

- Immunohistochemistry: positivity for desmin, myoglobin, MyoD1, skeletal muscle myogenin, sometimes also SMA.

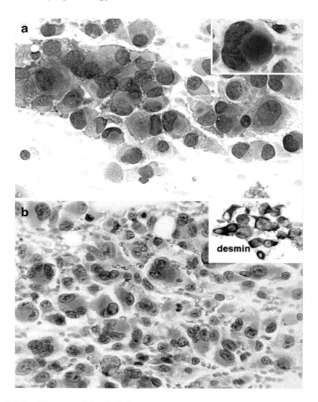

FIG. 6.10. *Pleomorphic rhabdomyosarcoma (PR)*: (**a**) The smears usually shows single cells among few tissue fragments. The cells are large, round, oval, and polygonal with obvious variation in size. (**b**) Numerous binucleated cells and multinucleated cells are also seen. Nuclei are hyperchromatic, eccentric, round with coarse chromatin, many irregularities of nuclear membrane and sometimes with prominent nucleoli. The Cytoplasm is abundant, well delineated and contains a globular structure in many cells.

Clear Cell Sarcoma (Fig. 6.11)

- A rare malignant tumor, known also as melanoma of soft parts, affecting mainly young adults aged between 30 and 40 years.
- Majority of tumors are located in the extremities, especially on the ankle and foot and are attached to tendons and fasciae.

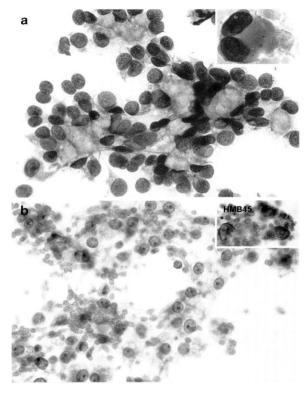

FIG. 6.11. *Clear cell sarcoma*: (**a**) The smears show predominance of single cells and few cell groups with microacinar cellular arrangement. The cells may be uniform or highly pleomorphic. Tumor cells are round, oval, and polygonal, sometimes admixed with few spindle cells as well as bi- and multinucleated cells. The cytoplasm is moderately abundant, some cells are vacuolated, individual cells may contain melanin. Nuclei are round or slightly oval and mainly positioned eccentrically, giving the cell a plasmacytoid shape. (**b**) Nuclei have single or multiple nucleoli and occasional cytoplasmic inclusions. The background can be lacy, vacuolated or tigroid and may contain bare nuclei or macrophages with melanin.

- Tumor grows slowly and some patients do not seek medical attention for years.
- Imaging data have benign characteristics.

- Prognosis is poor. Recurrence and metastatic rates are high; metastases can develop late in the course of disease.

Cytomorphology of Clear Cell Sarcoma

- Predominantly dissociated cells and few cell groups with loosely arranged cells. Microacinar cellular arrangement was also noticed.[40,41]
- The overall picture varies from unimorphous to highly pleomorphic.
- Tumor cells are round, oval, and polygonal, sometimes admixed with few spindle cells as well as bi- and multinucleated cells.
- Cytoplasm is moderately abundant, some cells are vacuolated, individual cells may contain melanin.
- Only rare cases are highly pigmented.[42]
- Nuclei are round or slightly oval and mainly positioned eccentrically, giving the cell a plasmacytoid shape. Nuclei have single or multiple nucleoli and occasional cytoplasmic inclusions.
- The background can be lacy, vacuolated or tigroid,[43] it can contain bare nuclei or macrophages with melanin.

Ancillary Studies

- Immunohistochemistry: positivity for HMB45, S100, and melan A.
- The majority of cases have a typical translocation t(12;22) (q13;q12).

Differential Diagnosis

- Metastatic melanoma and
- Carcinoma[41]
- Epithelioid variants of other sarcomas. In cytology, clear cell sarcoma is indistinguishable morphologically and immunocytochemically from metastatic melanoma.

Alveolar Soft Part Sarcoma (Fig. 6.12)

- An extremely rare malignant tumor which can occur at any age but is seen most frequently in older children and young adults.
- Most commonly reported locations are extremities in adults, and head and neck area in children.
- Tumor grows slowly, has a low recurrence rate but early and frequent metastases to the lungs, bones, and brain, which can be

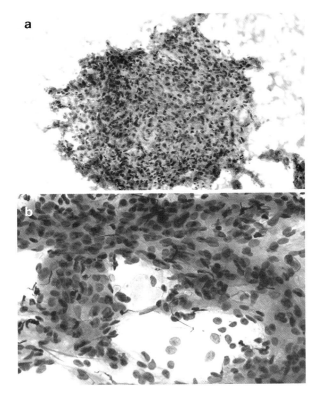

FIG. 6.12. *Alveolar soft part sarcoma*: (**a**) Cellular smears with single and cell groups of various size and naked nuclei. Tumor cells are large, polygonal, and round with abundant, fragile, granular cytoplasm and sometimes vacuolated at the periphery. Nuclei are large and centrally located with prominent nucleoli. Some cells are bi- and multinucleated. (**b**) Cell clusters can have a syncytial or pseudoacinar appearance. The background is usually hemorrhagic due to high vascularity of tumor or granular. It often contains many naked nuclei.

the first sign of disease. Sometimes metastases appear very late in the course of disease. The prognosis is poor.

Cytomorphology of Alveolar Soft Part Sarcoma

• Cellularity of smears reported in cytological literature is variable. There are cell groups of various size, dissociated cells, and naked nuclei.

- Tumor cells are large, polygonal, and round with abundant, fragile, granular cytoplasm and sometimes vacuolated at the periphery.
- The characteristic rod-shaped or rhomboid crystals seen in histology are rarely reported in cytological literature.[44]
- Nuclei are large and centrally located with prominent nucleoli. Some cells are bi- and multinucleated.[45]
- Cell clusters can have a syncytial[46] or pseudoacinar[47] appearance.
- Background is usually hemorrhagic due to high vascularity of tumor or granular. It often contains many naked nuclei.

Ancillary Studies

- Immunohistochemistry is not helpful because no consistent positivity for any antigens has been demonstrated.

Differential Diagnosis

- Granular cell tumor
- Rhabdomyoma,
- Paraganglioma,
- Renal cell carcinoma.

Synovial Sarcoma: Poorly Differentiated

A rare variant of poorly differentiated synovial sarcoma (PDSS) has large cells with moderately abundant cytoplasm and round nuclei with prominent nucleoli which sometimes lie eccentrically (plasmacytoid or rhabdoid appearance).[48]

Metastatic Tumors (Figs. 6.13–6.15)

- Metastases to soft tissues are uncommon as first manifestation of disease.
- Most commonly seen metastases in soft tissue are from carcinoma of the lung, breast, kidney, large bowel and from melanoma.
- Metastases of melanoma often appear many years after the removal of primary tumor, which may lead to the assumption that one is dealing with a new primary tumor.
- When samples are taken from retroperitoneal mass, primary tumors of adrenal gland, kidney, and pancreas must be considered

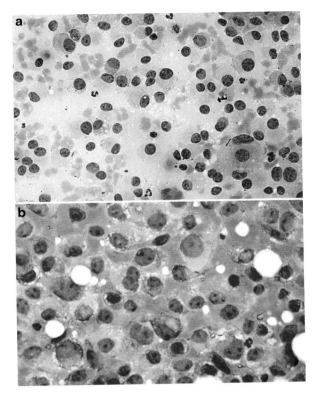

FIG. 6.13. *Metastatic carcinoma into soft tissue*: (**a**) Metastatic ader-enal cortical carcinoma: Large cells with abundant cytoplasm and eccentrically positioned nuclei. Giemsa, ×400. (**b**) Metastatic urothe-lial carcinoma: Polygonal cells with hyperchromatic nuclei, moderate anisonucleosis, prominent nucleoli, moderately abundant cytoplasm. Giemsa, ×60.

in the differential diagnosis with epithelioid-looking sarcomas. Imaging data cannot always point to the precise location of the original tumor.

- Liver metastases of sarcomas as well as primary hepatic sarco-mas may also cause problems to cytopathologists because they resemble metastatic carcinomas, which are far more common in this location.

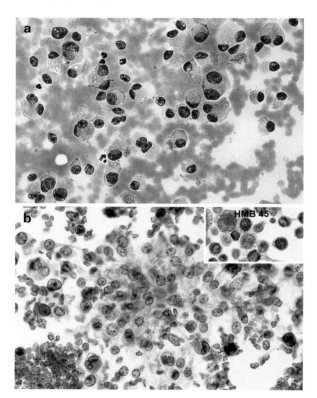

Fig. 6.14. *Metastatic melanoma*: (**a**) Cellular smears with numerous single cells. The cells are round, polygonal to spindle and some smears contain a mixture of all shapes. (**b**) The epithelioid or plasmacytoid morphology is common with abundant, well-demarcated cytoplasm, eccentric nuclei, many binucleated and multinucleated cells. Melanin is absent in positive immunohistochemical staining for HMB45 (insert), melan A and S-100 protein are useful markers except in differentiating melanoma from clear cell sarcoma.

Cytomorphology of Metastatic Tumors: Melanoma (Fig. 6.14)

- Smears from melanoma are highly cellular and contain mainly dissociated cells. Cell groups without organoid structure and accidental groupings are scarce or absent.

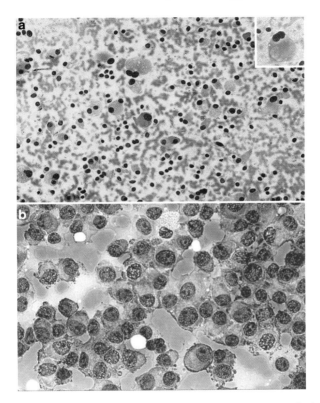

FIG. 6.15. (**a**) Metastatic medullary thyroid carcinoma into soft tissue: Plasmacytoid cells of various size, many naked nuclei. Giemsa, ×200. *Inset*: a large cell with two eccentric, small nuclei. Giemsa, ×400. (**b**) Metastatic breast carcinoma into soft tissue: Single cells with round, hyperchromatic nuclei, small nucleoli and abundant, well-delineated cytoplasm. Some cells are plasmacytoid. Giemsa, ×600.

- Morphology of melanoma varies greatly from round, polygonal to spindle and some smears contain a mixture of all shapes.
- Melanoma with epithelioid or plasmacytoid morphology is rather common: abundant, well-demarcated cytoplasm, eccentric nuclei, many binucleated, and multinucleated cells.
- Melanin is usually absent or present only in occasional cells.

- Positive immunocytochemical staining for HMB45, melan A, and S-100 protein are useful markers except in differentiating melanoma from clear cell sarcoma.

Cytomorphology of Metastatic Tumors: Carcinomas (Figs. 6.15a, b)

- Carcinoma of breast, lung, kidney (adeno and urothelial), adrenal gland, and medullary thyroid carcinoma can morphologically simulate sarcomas with epithelioid morphology. However, plasmacytoid morphology is not the only appearance of these tumors.
- In all above-mentioned carcinomas the common feature is predominance of dissociated cells which have a plasmacytoid appearance. Other features, like cell size, cytoplasmic staining and presence of vacuoles, binucleation, and nucleoli, vary somewhat within the same entity as well as between different entities.
- Immunohistochemistry: positivity for epithelial markers (except EMA in adrenal carcinomas). Medullary thyroid carcinoma expresses calcitonin, while many breast carcinomas express estrogen and progesterone receptors. TTF-1 is sometimes positive in lung carcinoma, namely adenocarcinomas.

Cytomorphology of Metastatic Tumors: Epithelial
Mesothelioma (Fig. 6.16)

- Predominantly dissociated cells and some clusters.
- Moderately large, round cells with eccentric, round nuclei and some binucleated cells. Some spindle cells can be mixed with round ones.
- Well-demarcated cytoplasm has vacuoles in some cells.
- Background can contain some myxoid substance.
- Tumor cells are positive for keratin, EMA, calretinin, HBME.

Lymphoma (Fig. 6.17)

- Non-Hodgkin lymphoma with an epithelioid appearance is mainly anaplastic large cell lymphoma (ALCL) and anaplastic variant of diffuse large B-cell (DLBC) lymphoma. Soft tissues may be the primary site of involvement in both lymphoma types.

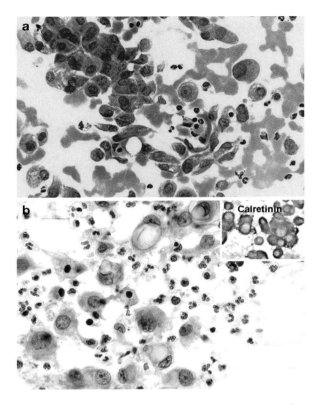

FIG. 6.16. *Metastatic epithelioid mesothelioma into soft tissue* of suprapubic region. (**a**) Dissociated, plasmacytoid and spindle cells and a group of cells with distinct boundaries. Giemsa, ×400. (**b**) Metastatic mesothelioma to the chest wall: Some cells have a lighter areas in the cytoplasm and others have vacuole simulating adenocarcinoma. Papanicolaou stain, ×600. *Inset*: positive calretinin on cytospin preparation, ×400.

- Extranodal presentation of Hodgkin lymphoma is rare, occurring in less than 5% of cases. The most common extranodal location is in the chest wall as the result of direct extension of the disease from anterior or posterior mediastinum.[49]
- Plasmacytomas may be found in soft tissue as the result of direct extension from lesions in bone, less commonly as solitary soft tissue lesions.

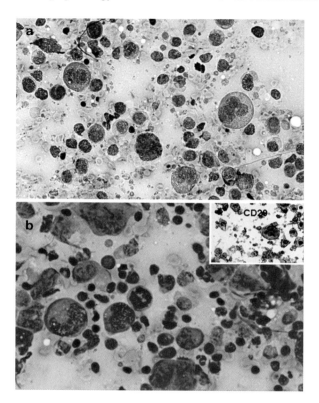

FIG. 6.17. *Non-Hodgkin's lymphoma*[49,50] with plasmacytoid cells in soft tissue: (**a** & **b**) Anaplastic variant of DLBCL featuring a mixed population of small and large, multinucleated tumor cells. Giemsa, ×400 and ×600. *Inset*: positive for CD20 on cytospin preparation. Non-Hodgkin's lymphoma with an epithelioid appearance is mainly anaplastic large cell lymphoma (ALCL) and anaplastic variant of diffuse large B-cell lymphoma. Soft tissues may be the primary site of involvement in both lymphoma types.

Cytomorphology of Non-Hodgkin Lymphoma with Epithelioid Cells

- Anaplastic variant of DLBC is made up of round and polygonal cells with one or more pleomorphic nuclei with nucleoli and moderate to abundant cytoplasm.

- Immunocytochemistry of anaplastic DLBC lymphoma: B-cell markers are positive as well as CD30. A panel of B-cell markers should be applied because some of them might be negative in individual cases.
- Smears from the common variant of ALCL contain moderate amount of large neoplastic cells, some of them bi- and multi-nucleated with prominent nucleoli (hallmark cells). Cytoplasm is abundant and often vacuolated. Tumor cells may appear in clusters. Background contains lymphocytes, eosinophils, histiocytes.
- In the small cell variant of ALCL diagnostic hallmark cells are rare and in the lymphohistiocytic variant hallmark cells can be obscured by histiocytes and plasma cells.

Ancillary Studies

- Immunocytochemistry of ALCL: hallmark cell are positive for CD30, ALK (60–85% of cases), EMA. There is variable positivity for LCA and T-cell antigens, CD2, and CD4 are most frequently positive.

Differential Diagnosis

- ALCL, anaplastic DLBC lymphoma and Hodgkin's lymphoma may not be differentiated on the basis of morphology. Immunocytochemistry is of great help except in the differential diagnosis between ALCL and Hodgkin's lymphoma where it can fail us. Carcinoma also comes into differential diagnosis.

Cytomorphology of Hodgkin Lymphoma

- Smears contain a reactive background consisting of lymphocytes, eosinophils, histiocytes, plasma cells, and variable number of tumor cells.
- The number of tumor cells is small in majority of cases but occasionally they can be numerous and therefore simulate ALCL, carcinoma, or sarcoma.
- Hodgkin cells are large, mononucleated with prominent nucleoli and moderate amount of cytoplasm. Reed–Sternberg cells are bi- and multinucleated, sometimes with a single nucleus which is multilobated. The number of tumor cells depends on the sub-type of Hodgkin lymphoma.

- In rare cases, smears may contain an abundance of neutrophils and thus simulate an inflammatory lesion.

Ancillary Studies

- Immunocytochemistry: In classical form tumor cells are positive for CD30, CD15 (75–85%) and CD20 (40%). In nodular

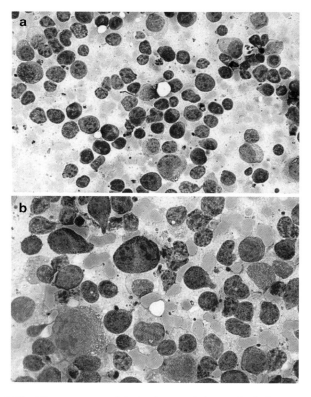

FIG. 6.18. *Plasmacytoma*: (**a**) A characteristic cytological appearance with mono and binucleated plasmacytoma cells, morphologically similar to plasma cells; Giemsa, ×400. (**b**) A rare anaplastic variant of plasmacytoma, simulating carcinoma or sarcoma; Giemsa stain, ×600. Rare anaplastic cases are pleomorphic and plasma cell origin is not recognizable morphologically. Immunocytochemistry: positivity for CD38 and CD138, restriction to α or κ light chains. Differential diagnosis includes melanoma, metastatic carcinomas and also sarcomas with plasmacytoid appearance.

lymphocyte predominant type tumor cells lack CD15 and CD30 and are positive for LCA and CD20.

Differential Diagnosis

- ALCL,
- Anaplastic DLBC,
- Metastatic carcinoma,
- Reactive lesions.

Cytomorphology of Plasmacytoma (Fig. 6.18)

- Smears are composed of completely dissociated cells which usually bear resemblance to plasma cells: round, eccentric nucleus with a cartwheel chromatin distribution and moderate amount of cytoplasm containing a lighter perinuclear zone.
- Anisocytosis is variable.
- Rare anaplastic cases are pleomorphic and plasma cell origin is not recognizable morphologically.

Ancillary Studies

- Immunocytochemistry: positivity for CD38 and CD138, restriction to κ or λ light chains.

Differential Diagnosis

- Melanoma,
- Metastatic carcinomas,
- Sarcomas with plasmacytoid appearance.

Tumors with Predominance of Round Cells

Rhabdomyosarcoma (Figs. 6.19 and 6.20)

- Rhabdomyosarcoma (RMS), a malignant tumor with muscle differentiation, is subdivided histologically into embryonal (including botryoid, spindle cell, and anaplastic variants) alveolar and pleomorphic subtypes.
- Embryonal and alveolar RMS is seen mainly in children and young adults and is rare in older patients. Pleomorphic RMS is a tumor of adults and does not belong to the round cell category.

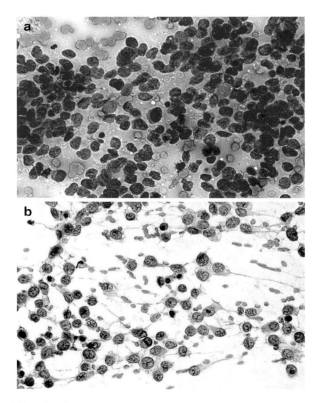

FIG. 6.19. *Alveolar rhabdomyoarcoma*: (**a**) Predominantly of small round blue cell tumor with naked nuclei and some preserved cells with high nuclear/cytoplasmic ratio. Nuclei are hyperchromatic, round, and somewhat irregular. Giemsa, ×600. (**b**) Irregularities of nuclear membrane and uneven chromatin distribution are well seen in Papanicolaou staining. (**c**) Highly cellular smear composed mainly of poorly organized cell groups (chance formations). Background is hemorrhagic. Giemsa, ×100. (**d**) Unimorphous population of round cells and chance formations. Naked nuclei prevail and only individual cells have moderate amount of poorly visible cytoplasm. Giemsa, ×400. (**e**) Hypechromatic nuclei with slight anisonucleosis. Only individual cells have preserved cytoplasm. Background is lacy (tigroid) and contains a few fat droplets. Giemsa, ×600. (**f**) A multinucleated tumor cell surrounded by a unimorphous population of rhabdomyoblasts. Giemsa, ×600. (**g**) Rhabdomyoblasts with many degenerative vacuoles. Giemsa, ×60. (**h**) Well-preserved rhabdomyoblasts with round nuclei which are placed eccentrically in moderate amount of cytoplasm. Tigroid background. Such a pattern with many mature rhabdomyoblasts is not a common finding. Giemsa, ×600. (**i**) Rhabdomyoblasts with high nuclear/cytoplasmic ratio, hyperchromasia and slight anisonucleosis. Giemsa, ×600; Papanicolaou, ×600.

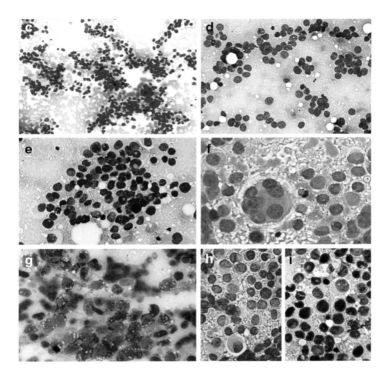

FIG. 6.19. (continued).

- In histology, only the alveolar RMS belongs to the small round cell category. In cytology, however, alveolar and embryonal RMS cannot always be separated and therefore embryonal RMS must also be considered in distinguishing between various round cell soft tissue tumors.
- Embryonal RMS is the most common variant, occurs in young children, most frequently in the head and neck region followed by urogenital region. It has a better prognosis than the alveolar RMS.
- Alveolar RMS occurs in older children, primarily on the extremities and in the paraspinal area.
- Prognostic factors in RMS include disease stage, tumor location and size, patient's age, and histologic subtype.

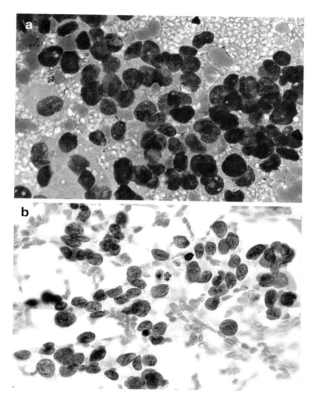

FIG. 6.20. *Embryonal rhabdomyoarcoma*: (**a**) Smears resemble different stages of skeletal muscle differentiation. It is generally less cellular that those from alveolar RMS. Predominate tumor cells are small, immature with uniform, slightly oval or round nuclei, while mature rhabdomyoblasts are rare. (**b**) Sometimes, embryonal RMS smears can be composed exclusively of dissociated, round cells with high nuclear/cytoplasmic ratio and are very similar to alveolar RMS.

Cytomorphology of Rhabdomyosarcoma: Alveolar (Fig. 6.19)

- Alveolar RMSs are highly cellular with predominantly dissociated cells and naked nuclei. Chance formations are seen in half of the cases (Fig. 6.19c, d) tissue fragments are seldom found and rarely contain small amount of eosinophilic stroma.
- Cells are round with high nuclear/cytoplasmic ratio (Fig. 6.19a, b, e)

- Nuclei are mostly round, hyperchromatic with nucleoli. Some nuclei are oval but these are seldom numerous. There is often slight anisonucleosis. The number of mature rhabdomyoblasts (plasmacytoid, tadpole or ribbon-shaped) varies from single to numerous (Fig. 6.19f, h) The same is true for binucleated and multinucleated cells (Fig. 6.19f). Mitotic figures are frequent.
- Cytoplasm is scant, often poorly delineated and difficult to see (Fig. 6.19a, e). It can contain small, degenerative vacuoles.[50] (Fig. 6.19g)
- Background may appear lacy or tigroid (Fig. 6.19e, f, h, i)

Ancillary Studies

- The majority of RMS are positive for desmin; however, this marker is not very specific. Myo D1 and myogenin are specific for RMS but MyoD1 is difficult to demonstrate.
- 75% of alveolar RMS have t(2;13)(q35;q14) translocation which can be demonstrated by FISH.

Differential Diagnosis

- Lymphoma,
- Ewing/PNET, desmoplastic small round cell tumor,
- Neuroblastoma,
- Malignant rhabdoid tumor.

Cytomorphology of Rhabdomyosarcoma: Embryonal (Fig. 6.20)

- Smears from embryonal RMS vary a great deal since this tumor resembles different stages of skeletal muscle differentiation.
- Smears from embryonal RMS are generally less cellular that those from alveolar RMS.
- Smears from the less differentiated areas contain some tissue fragments with moderate or abundant eosinophilic stroma which are moderately cellular.
- Tissue fragments without stroma are highly cellular.
- The number of dissociated cells among fragments is usually small but varies from single to numerous.[51]
- Predominate tumor cells are small, immature with uniform, slightly oval or round nuclei, while mature rhabdomyoblasts are rare.[52]

- Smears from the more mature areas of the tumor will show completely dissociated rhabdomyoblasts in various stages of maturation. In such cases there is greater variation of cell size and shape with plasmacytoid, tadpole, or strap-shaped cells as well as binucleated and multinucleated forms.
- Sometimes, embryonal RMS smears can be composed exclusively of dissociated, round cells with high nuclear/cytoplasmic ratio and are very similar to alveolar RMS.

Ancillary Studies

- The majority of RMS is positive for desmin; however, this marker is not very specific. Myo D1 and myogenin are specific for RMS but MyoD1 is difficult to demonstrate.

Differential Diagnosis

- Infantile myofibromatosis,
- Hemangioendothelioma and
- Neurofibroma due to stroma in tissue fragments.
- In cases with complete dissociation, which are inseparable from alveolar RMS, all other small round cell tumors must be considered.

Ewing Sarcoma/Primitive Neuroectodermal Tumor: PNET (Fig. 6.21)

- This family of tumors is more common in bones than in soft tissues.
- It occurs predominantly in children and young adults between ages 5 and 25.
- Since tumors are often painful and accompanied by fever, leukocytosis, and increased sedimentation rate, they are often mistaken for infections.
- Most common locations are extremities and chest wall. Bone tumors are often accompanied by a large soft tissue mass and are therefore easily aspirated.
- Bone lesions are osteolytic radiographically and have a moth-eaten appearance. Periosteal reaction produces a characteristic multilayered picture, referred to as "onion skin."
- Histologically, the Ewing sarcoma/PNET family of tumors includes morphologically diverse tumors which can be grouped

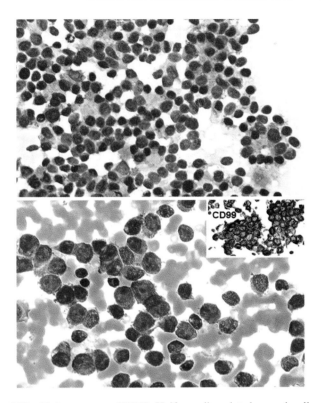

F{\scriptsize IG}. 6.21. *Ewing sarcoma/PNET*: Uniform dissociated, round cells and various number of rosette formations. Mixture of round and oval cells which vary slightly to moderately in size. Some cells have plasmacytoid shape and resemble rhabdomyoblasts. The cytoplasm is scant, sometimes well demarcated, in some smears it is poorly demarcated or absent in majority of cells. It can contain small degenerative vacuoles. Nuclei are round, hyperchromatic with slight to moderate anisonucleosis. Background can be lacy (tigroid).

  into typical Ewing sarcoma, adamantinoma-like, typical PNET, spindle cell variant, sclerosing, and large cell variants.[53]

- 85% of cases posses a t(11;22) (q24;q12) translocation which is helpful in identifying Ewing/PNET from other morphologically similar tumors.

- The overall survival is around 40%, depending on stage, tumor size, and location. When disease is metastatic upon discovery, survival is poor.[54]

Cytomorphology of Ewing/PNET

- Smears may contain only dissociated cells or a mixture of cell groups, dissociated cells, and naked nuclei.
- Cell groups are mostly chance formations, while tissue fragments and rosettes are less common. Some tissue fragments have stroma which stains pink in Giemsa.
- The most characteristic cytological picture, alas not the most common, is one composed almost entirely of monomorphous, dissociated, round cells, and various numbers of rosette formations.[55]
- The most commonly seen picture is a mixture of round and oval cells which vary slightly to moderately in size. Some cells have plasmacytoid shapes and resemble rhabdomyoblasts.
- Cytoplasm is scant, sometimes well demarcated, in some smears it is poorly demarcated or absent in a majority of cells.
- Cytoplasm can also contain small degenerative vacuoles.
- Nuclei are round, hyperchromatic with slight to moderate anisonucleosis.
- Rare cases have mostly oval nuclei and are indistinguishable morphologically and immunocytochemically from poorly differentiated synovial sarcomas since both tumors are positive for CD 99.
- Background can be lacy (tigroid), hemorrhagic, or it can contain cytoplasmic fragments simulating lymphoglandular bodies.

Ancillary Studies

- Majority of Ewing/PNET cases are positive for CD99; however, this marker is not specific since it can be demonstrated in various percentages in the majority of tumors that come into the differential diagnosis with Ewing/PNET (lymphoblastic lymphoma, neuroblastoma, RMS, DSRCT, synovial sarcoma.)
- Approximately 10% of Ewing/PNET cases are positive also for cytokeratin and desmin.

Differential Diagnosis

- Lymphoblastic lymphoma,
- Neuroblastoma,
- RMS,
- DSRCT,
- Synovial sarcoma.

Neuroblastoma (Fig. 6.22)

- Neuroblastoma is a malignant small round cell tumor of childhood (90% of cases occurring before the age of 5 years).

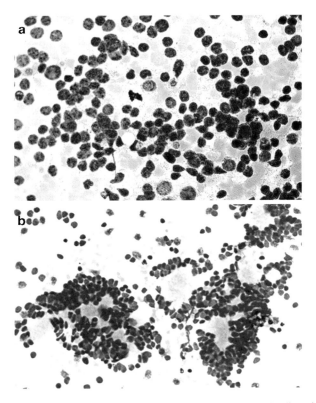

FIG. 6.22. *Neuroblastoma*: (**a**) Smears contain predominantly dissociated cells, few chance formations and various number of Homer–Wright rosettes. Nuclear molding is typical, producing small clusters and Indian files. Homer–Wright rosettes are formed by cells with nuclei arranged around a central area of fibrillary material made of cytoplasmic processes – neuropil. (**b**) Rosettes can be only rudimentary in poorly differentiated neuroblastomas. Sometimes pools of neuropil are also seen outside rosettes. Tumor cells have round, hyperchromatic nuclei, which are slightly irregular. Cytoplasm is scant or moderate. Some cells have slender cytoplasmic processes.

- Neuroblastoma originates in sympathetic ganglia and can be located anywhere in the para midline, most commonly in the retroperitoneum followed by the mediastinum, cervical, and pelvic regions.
- Patients with neuroblastoma appear chronically ill and present with fever, anemia, weight loss, and diarrhea in addition to symptoms associated with tumor location. Metastases in bones or lymph nodes may be the first presentation of disease.
- Majority of patients have elevated levels of catecholamines and their metabolites in the urine which is a helpful diagnostic tool.
- The most important favorable prognostic factors are patient's age lower than 2 years and low disease stage. Additional favorable factors are low number of N-myc amplifications, hyperdiploidy, low serum ferritin.
- Histologically neuroblastoma is subdivided into undifferentiated, poorly differentiated, and differentiating forms according to the percentage of cells showing differentiation into ganglion cells.

Cytomorphology of Neuroblastoma

- Cytomorphology of neuroblastoma depends on the degree of differentiation.
- Smears from differentiating and well-differentiated neuroblastoma contain predominantly dissociated cells, few chance formations and various number of Homer–Wright rosettes.
- Nuclear molding is typical, producing small clusters and single files of cells
- Homer–Wright rosettes are formed by cells with nuclei arranged around a central area of fibrillary material made of cytoplasmic processes – neuropil.[56]
- Rosettes can be only rudimentary in poorly differentiated neuroblastomas. Sometimes, pools of neuropil are also seen outside rosettes.
- Tumor cells have round, hyperchromatic nuclei, which are slightly irregular.
- Cytoplasm is scant or moderate. Some cells have slender cytoplasmic processes.
- The degree of anisonucleosis also varies with differentiation. In tumors differentiating toward ganglioneuroblastoma there is

clear pleomorphism with prominent anisonucleosis but without typical ganglion cells.

- Ganglion cells from ganglioneuroblastoma are large with abundant cytoplasm and prominent nucleoli. Some are binucleated and multinucleated. In ganglioneuroma, ganglion cells are mixed with neuronal fragments with spindle-shaped nuclei.
- Poorly differentiated neuroblastoma have no rosettes or neuropil. Cells are small with high nuclear/cytoplasmic ratios, containing uniform, round or slightly oval nuclei and are morphologically indistinguishable from undifferentiated blastema of Wilm's tumor (nephroblastoma), which is also located in the retroperitoneum.

Ancillary Studies

- Immunohistochemically neuroblastomas are positive for NB84 and CD56. These markers are not specific for neuroblastoma since they are positive also in other small round cell tumors.[57]

Differential Diagnosis

- Ewing/PNET, RMS desmoplastic small round cell tumor,
- Nephroblastoma, and lymphoma.

Desmoplastic Small Round Cell Tumor (Fig. 6.23)

- Desmoplastic small round cell tumor (DSRCT) is a rare neoplasm affecting predominantly males in the third decade, less commonly seen in younger and older patients.
- Retroperitoneum, omentum, and pelvis are most commonly affected; some cases have been reported also in the thorax and paratesticular area.
- Clinical symptoms include pain, accumulation of serosal fluid, organ obstruction.
- As the name implies, tumor is composed of abundant desmoplastic stroma containing variably sized nests of small neoplastic cells with focal areas of epithelial differentiation in the form of rosettes and even glandular structures. Stroma is highly vascularized.
- Prognosis of DSRCT is poor.

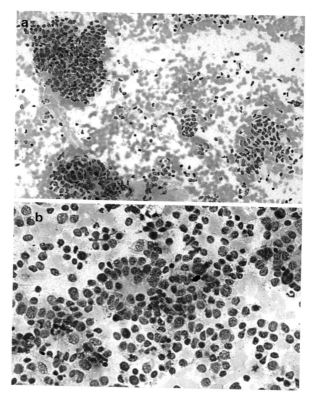

FIG. 6.23. *Desmoplastic small round cell tumor (DSRCT)*: (**a, b**) Smears are moderately or highly cellular, composed of cell groups and dissociated cells and occasional stromal fragments. Cell clusters can be loosely or tightly cohesive, sometimes in the form of sheets, tubules or well-formed rosettes. Stroma is acellular or contains a few fibroblasts and is intensely eosinophilic in Giemsa. Tumor cells have a high nuclear/cytoplasmic ratio, oval or round nuclei displaying slight to moderate anisonucleosis and sometimes small nucleoli. (**c**) Similar pattern as in (**a**) but with less stroma and some loosely and tightly arranged cell clusters. Giemsa, ×200. (**d**) A well-formed rosette mimicking the Homer–Wright rosette of neuroblastoma. Giemsa, ×400. (**e**) A smear composed predominantly of cells with round nuclei. Giemsa, ×600. (**f**) Two cell clusters as seen in the Papanicolaou staining. Papanicolaou, ×600.

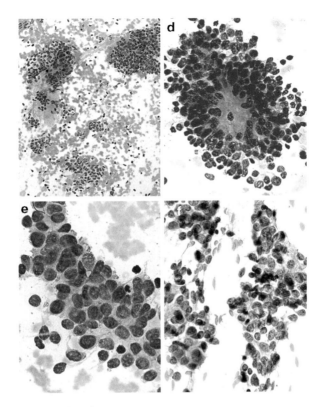

FIG. 6.23. (continued).

Cytomorphology of DSRCT

- Smears are moderately or highly cellular, composed of cell groups and dissociated cells while stromal fragments are not always present.[58]
- Cell groups are usually abundant while the number of dissociated cells varies a great deal.
- Cell clusters can be loosely or tightly cohesive (Fig. 6.23a–c) sometimes in the form of sheets, tubules, or well-formed rosettes.[59] (Fig. 6.23b, d)
- Stroma is acellular or contains a few fibroblasts and is intensely eosinophilic in Giemsa. It can be scant or abundant and clusters of tumor cells are tightly connected with it (Fig. 6.23b, d, e)

- Tumor cells have a high nuclear/cytoplasmic ratio, oval or round nuclei (Fig. 6.23e, f) displaying slight to moderate anisonucleosis and sometimes small nucleoli.[60]

Ancillary Studies

- A typical feature of DSRCT is its polyphenotypic differentiation, expressing epithelial, myogenic, and neural markers.[61] Tumor is positive for cytokeratin, epithelial membrane antigen (EMA), desmin, CD99, NSE, WT1(nuclear reaction).
- The specific genetic abnormality in DSRCT is the t(11;22) (p13;q12) translocation which is diagnostically useful.

Differential Diagnosis

- Ewing/PNET,
- RMS,
- Synovial sarcoma,
- Mesothelioma,
- Carcinoma.

Poorly Differentiated Synovial Sarcoma (with Round Cells) (Fig. 6.24)

Synovial sarcoma is primarily a spindle cell neoplasm which can be monophasic or biphasic, containing also an epithelial component.

- Poorly differentiated synovial sarcoma is less common. Three morphological variants are known: high-grade spindle type, epithelioid type with rhabdoid features and a round cell variant.
- Tumor location, immunohistochemistry, and genetic characteristics are the same as in regular synovial sarcoma.

Cytomorphology of Poorly Differentiated Synovial Sarcoma with Round Cells

- Smears are highly cellular containing dissociated cells, naked nuclei, and variable number of tissue fragments with tightly packed cells.
- Some tissue fragments may contain capillaries and rosette formations are also noted.[62]

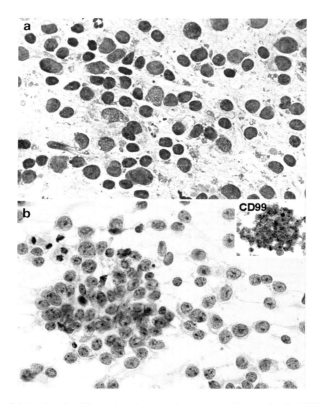

Fig. 6.24. *Poorly differentiated synovial sarcoma with round cells (PDSS)*:
(**a**) Smears are cellular with dissociated cells, naked nuclei and variable
number of tissue fragments with tightly packed cells with rosette formations. (**b**) Tumor cells have round and oval nuclei; each type of nuclear shape
may prevail. Nuclear/cytoplasmic ratio is high; sometimes mainly naked
nuclei are seen. Some cases will contain abundant eosinophilic stroma in
which tumor cells are embedded. Differential diagnosis includes mainly
Ewing/PNET and alveolar.

- Tumor cells have round and oval nuclei; either type of nuclear
  shape may prevail.
- Nuclear/cytoplasmic ratio is high; sometimes mainly naked
  nuclei are seen.
- Some cases will contain abundant eosinophilic stroma in which
  tumor cells are embedded.

Ancillary Studies

- Immunocytochemistry is of limited value especially in separating synovial sarcoma from Ewing/PNET. 32% of PDSS express CD99 while only 60% express cytokeratin.

Differential Diagnosis

- Ewing/PNET
- Alveolar rhabdomyosarcoma.

Extraskeletal Myxoid Chondrosarcoma (Fig. 6.25)

Cytomorphology of Extraskeletal Myxoid Chondrosarcoma (Cellular Variant)

- EMC is a tumor with a predominance of myxoid stroma. However, a variety of EMC, which is called a cellular variant (WHO), is hypercellular, containing little stroma.
- Tumor cells are large, epithelioid with abundant cytoplasm.
- Another cellular variant is composed of small round cells with a high nuclear/cytoplasmic ratio. This variant is similar to Ewing/PNET and poorly differentiated synovial sarcoma.

Paraganglioma (Fig. 6.26)

- A benign or malignant tumor of neural crest origin associated with autonomic ganglia.
- Three main locations include head and neck region, mediastinum, and retroperitoneum. The most common extrarenal paraganglioma is carotid body tumor.
- Patients with paragangliomas in retroperitoneum and posterior mediastinum are 30–45 years old; paragangliomas in other locations affect older patients (40–60 years).
- Radiographical images show high vascularity.
- Histological criteria of malignancy are not clear and metastases are the only definitive sign of a malignant lesion.

Cytomorphology of Paraganglioma

- Some smears are very cellular with tissue fragments and dissociated cells while those that are hemorrhagic contain only a few cell groups.

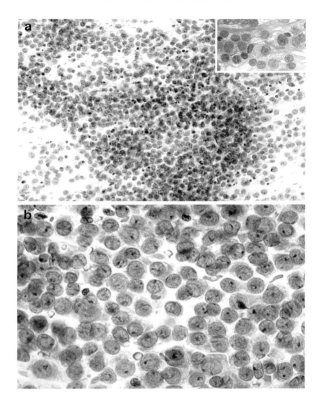

FIG. 6.25. *Extraskeletal myxoid chondrosarcoma (EMC);* (**a**) *cellular variant*: Hypercellular tumor containing little stroma. Tumor cell are large, epithelioid with abundant cytoplasm. (**b**) Another cellular variant is composed of small round cells with a high nuclear/cytoplasmic ratio. This variant is similar to Ewing/PNET and poorly differentiated synovial sarcoma.

- Cell groups are loosely arranged with occasional gland-like structures.
- Some tissue fragments are highly vascular.
- Stroma can also be seen occasionally.
- Cells are small or moderate in size with round and oval nuclei. The degree of anisonucleosis varies from monomorphous to moderately pleomorphic regardless of biological tumor potential.[63]
- Even in a monomorphous population there are often individual cells with markedly enlarged, hyperchromatic nuclei.

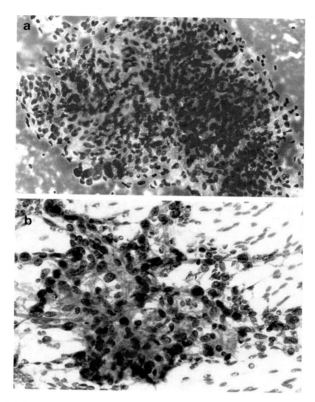

Fig. 6.26. *Paraganglioma*: (**a**) Smears are cellular with tissue fragments and dissociated cells while those that are hemorrhagic contain only a few cell groups. (**b**) Cell groups are loosely arranged with occasional gland-like structures. Some tissue fragments are highly vascular and stroma can also be seen occasionally. Cells are small or moderate in size with round and oval nuclei. The degree of anisonucleosis varies from uniform to moderately pleomorphic regardless of biological tumor potential. Cytoplasm is moderately abundant and poorly delineated. It can contain eosinophilic granula.

- Cytoplasm is moderately abundant and poorly delineated. It can contain eosinophilic granula.

Ancillary Studies

- Immunohistochemistry: positivity for NSE, chromogranin and synaptophysin.

Differential Diagnosis

- Medullary thyroid carcinoma, adenocarcinoma,
- Parathyroid tumors.

Glomus Tumor (Fig. 6.27)

- Glomus tumor is a rare entity derived from modified smooth muscle cells of glomus body.
- The principal locations are skin and superficial soft tissues of the extremities, namely subungual area, hand, foot. Many other locations have also been documented. Patients with glomus tumor are young or middle aged.
- The malignant glomus tumors are even less common than the benign ones and are usually located deeper.
- Superficially located glomus tumors are painful.

Cytomorphology of Glomus Tumor

- Cellularity of smears varies from scant to abundant, many smears are hemorrhagic.
- Cell clusters and dissociated cells are present but the number of each component is variable.
- In benign cases tumor cells are small, round with round nuclei of equal size. Cytoplasm is poorly demarcated.
- Background can contain myxoid material.[64]

Ancillary Studies

- Immunohistochemistry: positivity for smooth muscle actin.

Differential Diagnosis

- Epithelial neoplasms
- Epithelioid vascular tumors.

Solitary Fibrous Tumor (Fig. 6.28)

- An uncommon tumor affecting adults and occasionally children.
- It is located superficially and in deep soft tissues of various locations: extremities, head and neck, thoracic wall, retroperitoneum, mediastinum.
- Most cases are benign, some are malignant.

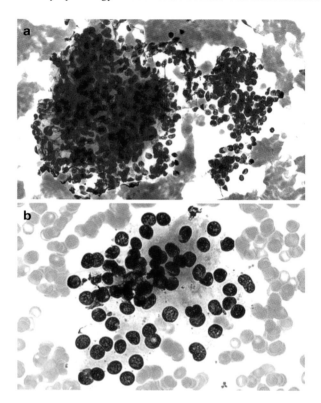

FIG. 6.27. *Glomus tumor*: (**a**) Cell clusters and dissociated cells are present but the number of each component is variable. (**b**) The tumor cells are small, round with round nuclei of equal size. Cytoplasm is poorly demarcated. Background can contain myxoid material.

- In histological sections there are hypocellular and hypercellular areas of small round and spindle cells, bands of hyalinized stroma and branching vascular spaces (hemangiopericytoma pattern).
- In malignant tumors there is high cellularity, numerous mitoses, necrosis, and atypia.

Cytomorphology of Solitary Fibrous Tumor

- Majority of solitary fibrous tumors are composed predominantly of spindle cells or they contain a mixture of spindle and round cells. However, some smears can be composed entirely of round cells.

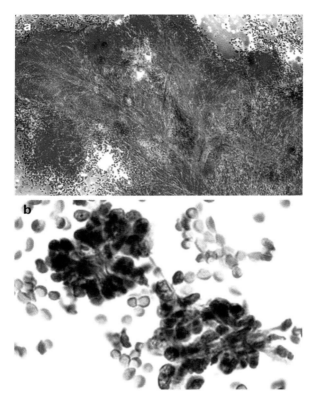

FIG. 6.28. *Solitary fibrous tumor*: (**a**) Most solitary fibrous tumors are composed predominantly of spindle cells or they contain a mixture of spindle and round cells. However, some smears can be composed entirely of round cells. (**b**) Cell groups, dissociated cells and naked nuclei are present in variable numbers. When larger tissue fragments are present they contain numerous capillaries. Tumor cells are round, medium sized with scant cytoplasm. Some cells appear plasmacytoid due to peripheral location of nuclei.

- Cell groups, dissociated cells and naked nuclei are present in variable numbers.
- When larger tissue fragments are present they contain numerous capillaries.
- Tumor cells are round, medium sized, monomorphous with scant cytoplasm. Some cells appear plasmacytoid due to peripheral location of nuclei.

Ancillary Studies

- Immunohistochemistry: positivity for CD34 and CD99 in majority of cases. EMA, BCL2, SMA and S100 may also be positive.

Differential Diagnosis

- It is not possible to separate benign solitary fibrous tumors from malignant ones because malignant tumors often lack atypia.

Non-Hodgkin Lymphomas (Fig. 6.29)

- Non-Hodgkin lymphomas may occasionally occur in soft tissues as primary manifestation of disease. The appearance of soft tissue lymphoma deposits at a later stage of disease is more common.
- B-cell lymphomas are more frequently found than peripheral T-cell lymphomas.
- The most commonly affected sites are extremities.

Cytomorphology of Non-Hodgkin Lymphomas

- Smears are usually very cellular containing completely dissociated cells.
- Cellular morphology depends a great deal on the type of lymphoma. Common features in most types are round cells, high nuclear cytoplasmic ratios, scant cytoplasm, many naked nuclei, and lymphoglandular bodies in the background.
- Variable features are cell size, degree of anisocytosis and anisonucleosis, presence and size of nucleoli.

Ancillary Studies

- Immunohistochemistry: positivity for LCA and other B- and T-cell antigens. Immunophenotyping with the aid of flow cytometer is very helpful.

Differential Diagnosis

- All small round cell tumors,
- Especially alveolar RMS,
- Ewing/PNET.

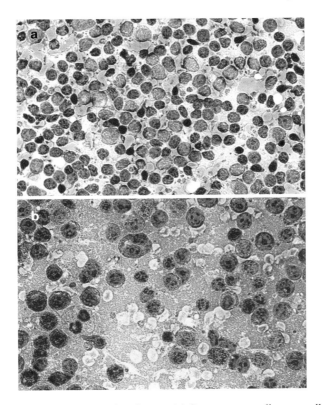

FIG. 6.29. *Non-Hodgkin's lymphomas*: (**a**) Smears are usually very cellular containing completely single cells. (**b**) The common features in most types are round cells, high nuclear cytoplasmic ratio, scant cytoplasm, many naked nuclei and lymphoglandular bodies in the background. Variable features are cell size, degree of anisocytosis and anisonucleosis, presence, and size of nucleoli.

Soft Tissue Lesions with Predominance of Inflammatory/Reactive Cells

Inflammation (Figs. 6.30–6.32)

- Soft tissues are rarely the primary site of inflammation caused by hematogenous spread of inflammatory agent. More commonly the inflammation spreads from the nearby skin, bone, or visceral lesions.

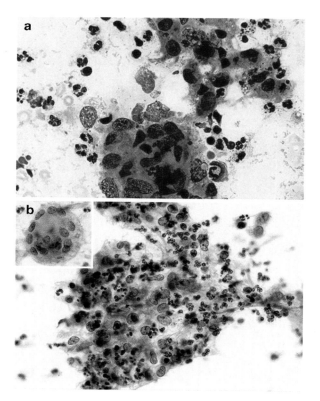

FIG. 6.30. *Acute inflammation in soft tissue*: (**a**) Histiocytes and reactive stromal cells in single and cell group with round, hyperchromatic nuclei, and moderately abundant cytoplasm which may contain debris. Numerous neutrophils in the background. Giemsa, ×40. (**b**) Histiocytes and reactive stromal cells in cell groups, simulating carcinoma, Papanicolaou, ×60. *Inset*: a multinucleated giant cell. Papanicolaou, ×60.

- Acute inflammation has a rapid onset, accompanied by pain in the affected part. Due to obvious clinical signs it is rarely mistaken for a neoplasm and seldom aspirated.
- Chronic inflammation has an insidious onset and runs a protracted course. Therefore neoplasm comes into the differential diagnosis.

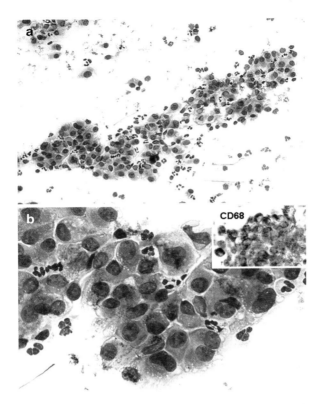

Fig. 6.31. *Granulomatous inflammation with predominance of histiocytes*: (**a**) A large group of histiocytes surrounded by some granulocytes. Giemsa stain, ×200. (**b**) Histiocytes have round shape, abundant cytoplasm and hyperchromatic nuclei, which are mostly positioned eccentrically and simulate malignant cells. Giemsa stain, ×600. *Inset*: positive immunocytochemical staining for CD68. Cytospin preparation, ×400.

- Chronic inflammation can be caused by infecting agents (bacteria, parasites, fungi) or by foreign bodies and chemicals. In some conditions cause is unknown (sarcoidosis).[65]

Cytomorphology of Inflammation

- In acute inflammation neutrophils predominate. Smears from an abscess have numerous, partly degenerated neutrophils mixed

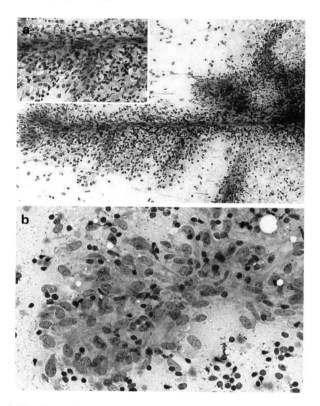

FIG. 6.32. *Granulation tissue formation and granulomatous inflammation*: (**a**) A fragment of granulation tissue with branching capillary network surrounded by histiocyte, lymphocytes and neutrophils. Giemsa stain, ×200. *Inset*: same at ×400. (**b**) Granulomatous inflammation with a group of epithelioid cells with oval and elongated nuclei and abundant cytoplasm surrounded by lymphocytes. Giemsa stain, ×400.

with fibrin and some macrophages with ingested debris in their cytoplasm.

- The main cells in chronic inflammation are lymphocytes, histiocytes, and fibroblasts accompanied by neutrophils, eosinophils, plasma cells, and macrophages.
- Histiocytes have round or bean-shaped nuclei and moderate amounts of cytoplasm. Special type of histiocytes are epithelioid cells and multinucleated giant cells.

- Epithelioid cells are found in granulomas.[66] They usually appear in clusters, have oval or round nuclei and abundant cytoplasm. They can be mistaken for carcinoma cells.
- Multinucleated giant cells are fused histiocytes. According to the arrangement of nuclei they are called foreign body, Touton, or Langhans giant cells (Fig. 6.31).
- Smears from chronic inflammation may contain parts of granulation tissue which forms due to healing process around the inflamed area. It is made of blood vessels, myofibroblasts, and histiocytes (Fig. 6.32a).

Fasciitis/Myositis (Fig. 6.33)

- Proliferative fasciitis is a rapidly growing but self-limiting process seen most commonly on the upper extremities, thorax, and neck of young adults.
- Proliferative myositis is more common in patients over 45 years of age. It is found in the muscles of shoulder, thorax and thigh. Unlike proliferative fasciitis it does not appear as a tumor but as an induration which is ill-defined.
- Both conditions have been also described in children where the initial histologic diagnosis was sarcoma in high percentage.[67]
- Common to both conditions is the fact that they can be mistaken for sarcoma microscopically due to presence of large, ganglion-like cells which resemble rhabdomyoblasts.
- Focal myositis affects children and adults and gives clinically an impression of a neoplasm. The swelling is painful, growing slowly over the course of a few weeks, most commonly in the lower extremities.

Cytomorphology of Fasciitis/Myositis

- In proliferative fasciitis/myositis there are many dissociated cells, naked nuclei and tissue fragments; cases of myositis also have many fragments of partially degenerated muscle.
- Dissociated cells are fibroblasts and myofibroblasts. The latter are large or medium sized, polygonal, round, sometimes with cytoplasmic extensions. Nuclei are round, often positioned eccentrically. Some of these cells are very large with prominent nucleoli (ganglion-like cells).

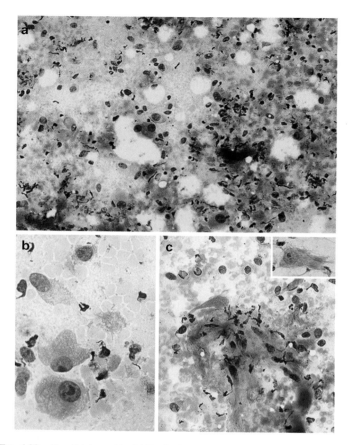

FIG. 6.33. *Fasciitis/myositis*: (**a**) Partly degenerated muscle fibers (*blue blobs*), many naked nuclei and scattered myofibroblasts (ganglion-like cells). Giemsa stain, ×100. (**b**) Myofibroblasts are large cells with abundant cytoplasm and round nucleus, which is often located at the periphery of the cell. Nuclei contain prominent nucleoli. Giemsa stain, ×600. *Inset*: Myofibroblasts look smaller in Papanicolaou staining due to alcohol fixation. (**c**) A stromal fragment, some degenerated muscle fibers, and fibrocytes and fibroblasts. Giemsa stain, ×400.

- Tissue fragments have eosinophilic stroma and variable numbers of stromal cells.
- In focal myositis, lymphocytes are the predominant inflammatory cells accompanied by neutrophils, plasma cells, and macrophages.

Smears also contain fragments of degenerated muscle and elements of muscle regeneration.[68]

Differential Diagnosis

- Differential diagnosis includes sarcomas with similar rhabdomyoblast-like cells.

Fat Necrosis (Fig. 6.34)

- It is a benign condition usually caused by trauma.

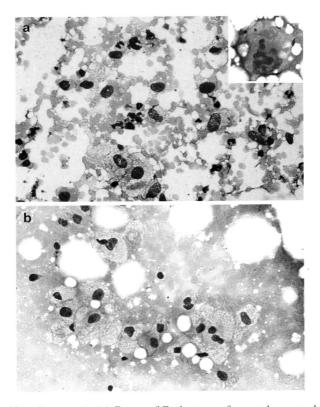

FIG. 6.34. *Fat necrosis*: (**a**) Groups of Coalescence of macrophages produces multinucleated syncytial forms. Giemsa, ×600. (**b**) The lipophages have foamy cytoplasm and round or oval nuclei with mild anisonucleosis. Giemsa, ×400.

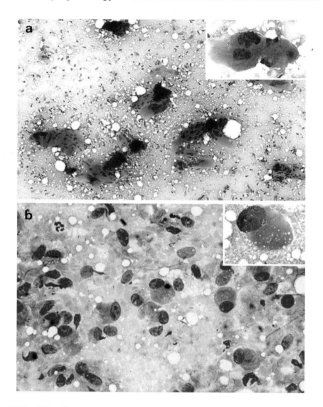

Fig. 6.35. *Muscle regeneration and repair:* FNA from a tumor-like reactive lesion on the neck of a child which appeared after blunt trauma. (**a**) Multinucleated, regenerating muscle cells. Thin, parallel lines in the cytoplasm represent partly formed myofibrils. Giemsa stain, ×100. *Inset*: a multinucleated regenerating muscle fiber. (**b**) Reactive mesenchymal cells, probably myofibroblasts are plasmacytoid and polygonal, simulating sarcoma. Giemsa, ×400. *Inset*: a reactive mesenchymal cell with rhabdoid appearance.

- Cytopathologists see fat necrosis predominantly in breasts after surgery or blunt trauma. The second most common location is in the gluteal area following repeated injections.
- In breast, fat necrosis simulates carcinoma clinically due to the presence of a firm lump with skin retraction. Radiological features may also be suspicious for malignancy.[69,70]

49. Khalbuss WE, Grigorian S, Mignone J, D'Agostino HJ. Chest wall abscesses: An unusual presentation of Hodgkin's lymphoma. *Diagn Cytopathol.* 2005;33:33–35.
50. Jiménez-Heffernan JA, Vicandi B, López-Ferrer P, Hardisson D, Viguer JM. Value of fine needle aspiration cytology in the initial diagnosis of Hodgkin's lymphoma. Analysis of 188 cases with an emphasis on diagnostic pitfalls. *Acta Cytol.* 2001;45:300–306.
51. Atahan S, Aksu Ö, Ekinci C. Cytologic diagnosis and subtyping of rhabdomyosarcoma. *Cytopathol.* 1998;9:389–97.
52. Pohar Marinšek Ž, Bračko M. Rhabdomyosarcoma: Cytomorfology, subtyping and differential diagnostic dilemmas. *Acta Cytol.* 2000;44: 524–532.
53. Kilijanienko J, Caillaud J-M, Orbach D, et al. Cyto-histological correlation in primary, recurrent and metastatic rhabdomyosarcoma: The Institute Curie's experience. *Diagn Cytopathol.* 2007;35:482–487.
54. Folpe AL, Goldblum JR, Rubin BP, Shehata BM, Liu W. Dei Tos AP, Weiss SW. Morphologic and immunophenotypic diversity in Ewing family tumors. *Am J Surg Pathol.* 2005;29:1025–1033.
55. Pohar Marinsek Ž, Kavalar R, Jereb B. Ewing sarcoma/PNET: 27 years of experience in Slovenia. *Ped Hematol Oncol.* 2006;23:355–367
56. Fröstad B, Tani E, Brosjö O, Skoog L, Kogner P. Fine needle aspiration cytology in the diagnosis and management of children and adolescents with Ewing sarcoma and peripheral primitive neuroectodermal tumor. *Med Pediatr Oncol.* 2002;38:33–40.
57. Pohar Marinsek Ž. Difficulties in diagnosig small roud cell tumours of childhood from fine needle aspiration cytology samples. *Cytopathol.* 2008;19:67–79.
58. Geisinger KR, Silverman JF, WakelyPE Jr. Neuroblastoma. In: Johnston WWJ, ed. *Pediatric cytopathology. ASCP theory and practice of cytopathology 4.* Chicago: ASCP Press; 1994:307–312.
59. Khalbuss WE, Bui M, Loya A. A 19-year-old woman with a cervicovaginal mass and elevated serum CA 125. Desmoplastic small round cell tumor. *Arch Pathol Lab Med.* 2006;130:e59–61.
60. Crapanzano JP, Cardillo M, Lin O, Zakowski MF. Cytology of desmoplastic small round cell tumor. *Cancer.* 2002;96:21–31.
61. Dave B, Shet T, Chinoy R. Desmoplastic round cell tumor of childhood: can cytology with immunocytochemistry serve as an alternative for tissue diagnosis? *Diagn Cytopathol.* 2005;32:330–5.
62. Granja NM, Begnami MD, Bortolan J, Filho AL. Schmitt FC Desmoplastic small round cell tumour: Cytological and immunocytochemical features. *Cytojournal.* 2005;2:6.
63. Akerman M, Domanski HA. The complex cytological features of synovial sarcoma in fine needle aspirates, an analysis of four illustrative cases. *Cytopathology.* 2007;18:234–40.

64. Zaharopoulos P. Diagnostic challenges in the fine-needle aspiration diagnosis of carotid body paragangliomas: report of two cases. *Diagn Cytopathol*. 2000;23:202–7.
65. Handa U, Palta A, Mohan H, Punia RP. Aspiration cytology of glomus tumor: a case report. *Acta Cytol*. 2001;45:1073–6.
66. Yamamoto T, Nagira K, Akisue T, et al. Aspiration biopsy of nodular sarcoidosis of the muscle. *Diagn Cytopathol*. 2002;26:109–12.
67. Guo M, Lemos L, Baliga M. Nodular sarcoid myositis of skeletal muscle diagnosed by fine needle aspiration biopsy. A case report. *Acta Cytol*. 1999;43:1171–6.
68. Meis JM, Enzinger FM. Proliferative fasciitis and myositis of childhood. *Am J Surg Pathol*. 1992;16:364–72.
69. Pinto Blázquez J, Velasco Alonso J, Menendez CL, Alonso de la Campa J, Astudillo. Fine needle aspiration cytology of focal myositis: a case report. *Acta Cytol*. 2005;49:653–655.
70. Aqel NM, Howard A, Collier DS. Fat necrosis of the breast: a cytological and clinical study. *Breast*. 2001;10:342–5.

7
Cytopathology of Adipocytic Soft Tissue Tumors

Živa Pohar-Marinšek[1] and Walid E. Khalbuss[2]

[1] Department of Cytopathology, Institute of Oncology, Ljubljana, Slovenia, EU

[2] University of Pittsburgh Medical Center, UPMC-Shadyside, POB2, Suite 201 Cytology, 5150 Centre Avenue, Pittsburgh, PA 15232, USA

Introduction

The most recent WHO classification of soft tissue tumors recognizes the following adipocytic tumors: lipoma, lipomatosis, lipomatosis of nerve, lipoblastoma, angiolipoma, myolipoma of soft tissue, chondroid lipoma, spindle cell lipoma/pleomorphic lipoma, hibernoma, atypical lipomatous tumor/well-differentiated liposarcoma (ALT/WDL), dedifferentiated liposarcoma, myxoid liposarcoma, pleomorphic liposarcoma, and mixed-type liposarcoma.[1]

In keeping with the concept of this book which classifies soft tissue tumors according to morphology, we can divide adipocytic tumors into the following categories:

1. *Fat resembling*: Lipoma, fibrolipoma, chondrolipoma, intramuscular lipoma, angiolipoma, hibernoma, lipoblastoma, and well-differentiated lipoblastoma
2. *Spindle cell*: Spindle cell lipoma and spindle cell variant of well-differentiated lipoblastoma
3. *Myxoid*: Myxoid liposarcoma

W.E. Khalbuss and A.V. Parwani, *Cytopathology of Soft Tissue and Bone Lesions*, Essentials in Cytopathology 9, DOI 10.1007/978-1-4419-6499-1_7,
© Springer Science+Business Media, LLC 2011

4. *Round cell*: Round cell liposarcoma
5. *Pleomorphic*: Pleomorphic lipoma, pleomorphic liposarcoma, and dedifferentiated liposarcoma

Since there is considerable variability within each class of adipocytic tumors it is not possible to make a perfect morphological separation into the above five categories and there is some overlap between them. For example, myxomatous degeneration of stroma is very common in adipocytic tumors and therefore many entities share characteristics with those in the myxoid group of lesions.

Adipocytic Tumors Resembling Fat

Lipoma NOS (Figs. 7.1–7.5)

- Lipoma is the most common soft tissue neoplasm, occurring mainly in adults between ages 40 and 60.
- Subcutaneous lipomas are exophytic, well demarcated, and soft on palpation; intramuscular lipomas appear more firm and less well demarcated, especially the infiltrating type.
- Radiological features are the same in lipomas as in the surrounding adipose tissue.
- Intramuscular infiltrating lipomas recur if wide excisional margins are not employed.
- In cytology, lipomas are morphologically indistinguishable from subcutaneous fat. Therefore, a definitive diagnosis of lipoma cannot be made on the basis of morphology alone. It is advisable to report that the material obtained is consistent with the clinical impression of lipoma when cytopathologist is confident that the material is representative. Otherwise one should state that specimen contains mature fat tissue, adding that lipoma cannot be confidently identified from subcutaneous fat.[2,3]

Cytomorphology of Lipoma

- Cellularity of smears from pure lipomas is variable and the yield is rarely abundant. Unsatisfactory smears are not unusual even in experienced hands from tumors that are easily sampled. Fat that is seen macroscopically at aspiration can be lost during

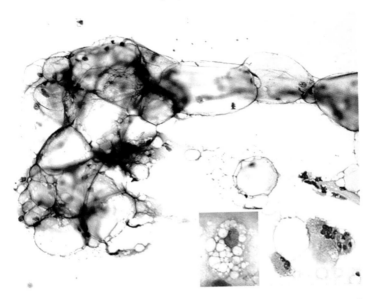

FIG. 7.1. **Lipoma FNA**: Smear from classic lipoma shows a cluster of mature lipocytes and a single lipocyte surrounded by free fat globules. (DQ, ×200). In the Inset (*left*) a multivacuolated cell from pure lipoma can resemble a lipoblast. In inset (*right*) multinucleated histiocytes are the result of degenerative changes in lipoma.

sample preparation and such smears contain many round empty spaces previously occupied by free fat globules.

- The most common findings in adequate samples are tissue fragments of variable size, composed of mature adipocytes and sometimes also capillary fragments. Single adipocytes are seen occasionally and are never abundant.
- Adipocytes are large, round cells varying somewhat in size, with well-delineated, empty cytoplasm and small, round nuclei at the periphery (Fig. 7.1). The cell membrane is often wrinkled (Fig. 7.1). Some adipocytes have many vacuoles and appear foamy. Free fat globules are intermixed with tissue fragments and it is not always possible to distinguish whether vacuoles are inside or outside the cell and can simulate lipoblasts (Fig. 7.1).

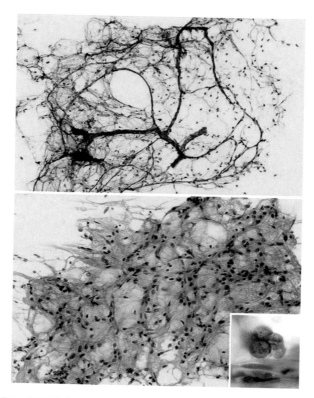

Fig. 7.2. **Pitfalls in Lipoma FNA**: *Upper*: A fragment from pure lipoma with extensive capillary network. There are vessels with narrow and wide lumens. (DQ stain, ×100). *Lower*: When many capillaries are present in pure lipoma, tissue fragments look cellular and simulate angiolipoma, spindle cell lipoma or ALT/WDL. (Pap stain, ×200). In the inset: a small cluster of atypical cells with enlarged nuclei.

- Capillary fragments are single or they form a small network. The diameter of blood vessels varies from narrow to middle size (Fig. 7.2).
- Tissue fragments with extensive capillary network appear densely cellular due to many oval nuclei of endothelial cells and simulate angiolipoma or spindle cell lipoma (Fig. 7.2).
- The background can be clear, hemorrhagic and/or can contain free fat globules in various quantities.

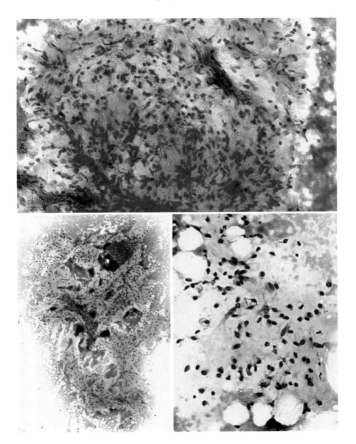

FIG. 7.3. **FNA of Fibrolipoma**: *Upper*: A very cellular tissue fragment from fibrolipoma contains a capillary and many fibrocytes and fibroblasts. Some oval nuclei belong to endothelial cells. The background is hemorrhagic. (DQ stain, ×200). *Lower left*: A stromal fragment from fibrolipoma is intensly eosinophilic (DQ stain, ×100). *Lower right*: A smaller, less cellular fragment from fibrolipoma amidst some free fat globules. Scattered cells are fibrocytes and fibroblasts. (DQ stain, ×200).

- Rare findings are small stromal fragments, mononuclear or multinuclear histiocytes (Fig. 7.1, inset), naked nuclei, and atypical cells (Fig. 7.1). The atypical nuclei are two to three times bigger than adipocytic nuclei and may be lobulated, probably

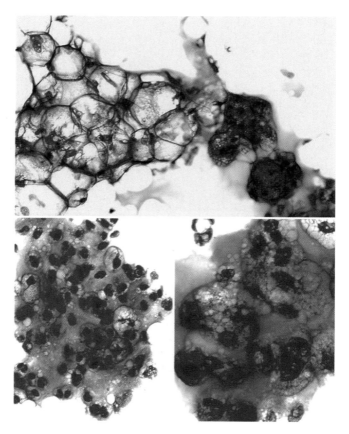

Fig. 7.4. **FNA of Chondroid Lipoma**: A tissue fragment from chondroid lipoma with adipocytes, stroma and lipoblasts. (DQ stain, ×400). The chondroid stroma is blue-violet (×400, *left*), and the myxoid stroma is intensly eosinophilic on DQ stain, ×600).

derived from areas of degenerative changes, the same as histiocytes. Such cases cannot be confidently distinguished from an ALT/WDL.

Differential Diagnosis

- Subcutaneous fat,
- Angiolipoma,

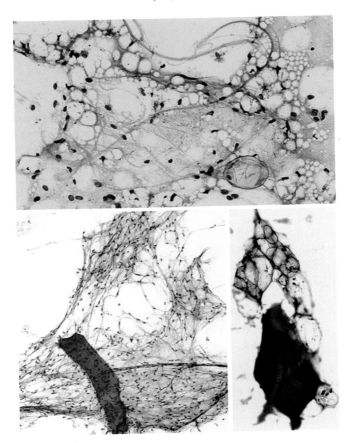

Fɪɢ. 7.5. **FNA of Intramuscular Lipoma.** *Upper:* Few stromal fragments in myxoid background containing fat droplets, some adipocytes and scattered cells with round, plasmacytoid or stellate appearance. (DQ stain, ×200). *Lower left:* A tissue fragment from intramuscular lipoma contains a fragment of striated muscle and moderate number of capillaries. Adipocytes are seen in the middle of the image. In Pap stained smear, muscle fibers and wider capillaries stain red. (Pap stain, ×100). *Lower right:* Muscle fibers stain blue in DQ stain, adipocytes are nicely visable. (DQ stain, ×200).

- Spindle cell lipoma,
- ALT/WDL.

Variants of Lipoma

Variants of lipoma can be classified into two categories:

(a) Lipomas with an admixture of other mesenchymal elements (osteolipoma, chondrolipoma, fibrolipoma, and myxolipoma).
(b) Lipomas of special locations (intramuscular lipoma, synovial lipoma).

- *Osteolipoma*: Representative samples cannot be aspirated because thin needle cannot penetrate the boney part of the tumor. Smears will look the same as those from pure lipomas.

- *Fibrolipoma*: In addition to adipocytes there are fragments of fibrous tissue which can be closely associated with adipocytic fragments or lie independently. The stroma is basophilic or intensely eosinophilic (Fig. 7.3) in Giemsa-stained smears while cellularity varies from sparse to moderate (Fig. 7.3) When only stromal fragments are sampled, smears resemble a fibroblastic tumor.

- *Chondrolipoma* (Fig. 7.4): Contains adipocytes and fragments of cartilage tissue. They have to be distinguished from chondroid lipomas which contain chondromatous stroma and lipoblasts but no true chondrocytes or chondroblasts.[4]

- *Myxolipoma*: Is a lipoma with myxoid degeneration of stroma. Smears contain adipocytes and various amounts of myxoid material. When myxoid material predominates, other benign or low-grade malignant tumors come into the differential diagnosis: spindle cell lipoma and hibernoma with myxoid change, myxoma, low-grade myxofibrosarcoma, fibromyxosarcoma.

- *Intramuscular lipoma*: Usually contains fragments of striated muscle which lie separately or in contact with adipocytic fragments (Fig. 7.5). Presence of muscle fragments is not an absolute indication of intramuscular lipoma since the same can be seen when striated muscle is sampled together with an adjacent pure lipoma. Many cases will contain myxoid stromal fragments with stellate, round or plasmacytoid cells, and an occasional adipocyte (Fig. 7.5). Such fragments can predominate and adipocytic nature cannot be recognized.

Angiolipoma (Fig. 7.6)

- Angiolipomas are common, benign subcutaneous tumors, single or multiple, located usually on forearm, less often on trunk and upper arm.
- They are often somewhat painful on palpation.
- First appearance in late teens or early 20s, more common in males.

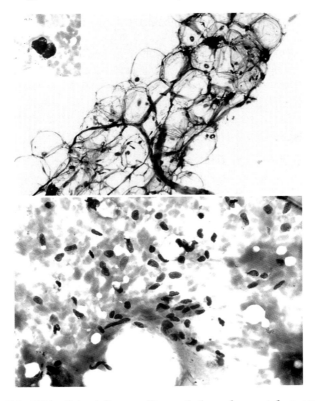

Fig. 7.6. **FNA of Angiolipoma**: *Upper*: A tissue fragment from angiolipoma with lipocytes and capillaries, similar to pure lipoma. (DQ, ×200). Inset shows two mastocytes. *Lower*: Smear from angiolipoma contains only a few areas with oval and spindle cells. (DQ stain, ×400).

Cytomorphology of Angiolipoma

- In cytology angiolipomas can seldom be separated from lipomas NOS, since the abundant capillary network, which distinguishes angiolipomas from classical lipomas in histology, is not represented in FNAB samples to such an extent that the difference could be appreciated.
- Fragments of adipocytes with thin and thick vascular fragments are present (Fig. 7.6). Some fragments appear very cellular and are similar to those from fibrolipoma (Fig. 7.6).
- An alternative pattern contains moderate number of cells with oval or spindle nuclei accompanied by few adipocytic fragments (Fig. 7.6).
- A few mastocytes may be present (Fig. 7.6, inset).
- Angiolipomas which undergo degenerative changes will contain a few histiocytes and other reactive cells and their naked nuclei which may appear slightly atypical.

Differential Diagnosis

- Same as in lipoma NOS.

Chondroid Lipoma (Fig. 7.4)

- Chondroid lipomas are rare benign tumors of adults, more common in females.
- They are located deeply in the subcutis or more often in muscles or connective tissues in arms and legs or limb girdles.

Cytomorphology of Chondroid Lipoma

- Fragments contain adipocytes as well as groups of lipoblasts embedded in stroma (Fig. 7.4) which can be chondroid (Fig. 7.4), collagenized (Fig. 7.4), or myxoid.
- Lipoblasts are smaller than mature adipocytes, show slight variation in size and have multi vacuolated cytoplasm.
- Cytoplasmic vacuoles of lipoblasts are small and even-sized or vary in size. Nuclei are medium sized, round, often lobulated (Fig. 7.4).

Differential Diagnosis

- Subcutaneous fat,
- Angiolipoma,
- Spindle cell lipoma,
- ALT/WDL.

Hibernoma (Fig. 7.7)

- Hibernomas are rare benign tumors which are a combination of brown fat and white adipose tissue.
- They occur at all ages but are most frequently seen in young adults.
- A variety of locations have been reported, most commonly in thigh and back, lying in subcutis or intramuscularly. Intra-abdominal and mediastinal locations are also possible.
- Imaging features do not have characteristics of an adipocytic tumor.
- There are six histological variants of hibernoma based on morphology of brown fat, capillary content, and the appearance of stroma: eosinophilic, pale cell, mixed, lipoma-like, myxoid, spindle cell.

Cytomorphology of Hibernoma

- A moderate number of tissue fragments which resemble those from lipoma at low power; however, cells are multivacuolated (Fig. 7.7).
- Many cell clusters contain capillary fragments, sometimes quite numerous.
- Large cells have many small, uniform vacuoles and centrally positioned small nuclei (Fig. 7.7).
- Some cells are not vacuolated and look granular.
- In the pale variant vacuoles are larger and vary in size; in the mixed variant both types of vacuolated cells are present.
- Smears from the lipoma-like variant contain clusters of uni-vacuolated adipocytes and clusters of multivacuolated brown fat cells.

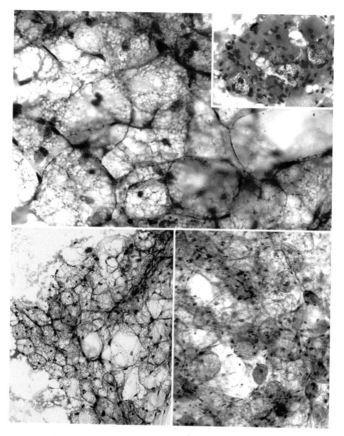

Fig. 7.7. **FNA of Hibernoma**: *Upper*: Image at high power with many small, uniform vacuoles in the cytoplasm and some capillary fragments between cells. (DQ stain, ×400). Insert: A group of granular cells. (DQ stain, ×400). *Lower*: The morphology resembles pure lipoma (*left*, DQ stain, ×200, *right*, Pap stain, ×200).

- The background is hemorrhagic and often contains free fat globules. Myxoid material is present in rare myxoid variants.
- The spindle cell variant is a combination of hibernoma and spindle cell lipoma which cannot be recognized in cytology unless both components are sampled.

Differential Diagnosis

- Mainly lipoma NOS and liposarcoma.
- Granular cell tumor and rhabdomyoma must be excluded in case of many granular cells.[5]

Lipoblastoma (Fig. 7.8)

- Lipoblastomas are benign tumors of childhood, occurring mainly during the first 3 years of life, which resemble fetal adipose tissue.
- They are more common in boys and have predilection for extremities but many other locations have been reported.
- Radiological features are similar to those of other adipocytic tumors.
- Recurrences are frequent in the diffuse type (lipoblastomatosis) and have to be excised with wide margins.
- Lipoblastomas contain mature adipocytes and lipoblasts in various stages of maturation including immature mesenchymal cells. The number of individual cell types and the amount of myxoid change varies. Therefore one can also expect variability in cytological pictures.

Cytomorphology of Lipoblastoma

- Smears from lipoblastomas contain a moderate number of tissue fragments with myxoid stroma, extensive plexiform vascular pattern, numerous, small cells with oval nuclei, and univacuolated adipocytes.[6,7]
- Some fragments contain a mixture of adipocytes and multivacuolated lipoblasts. The proportion of adipocytes and lipoblasts varies from case to case (numerous adipocytes and few lipoblasts [8] or vice versa).[9]
- Background can contain abundant myxoid material and/or many fat droplets.[10]
- Nuclei of adipocytes and multivacuolated lipoblasts are small and uniform while the oval nuclei of spindle cells are plump, bland, uniform (Fig. 7.8) in some cases or show moderate degree of atypia in others. Their cytoplasm is scant.

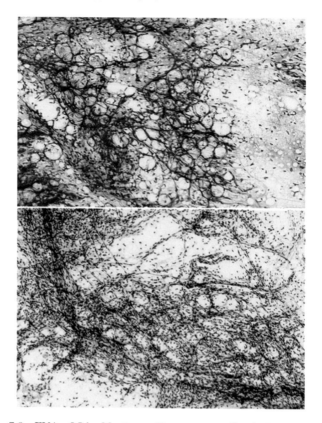

FIG. 7.8. **FNA of Lipoblastoma**: Numerous small spindle cells, abundant capillary network and few adipocytes in abundant myxoid stroma. (DQ stain, ×100, *Upper*, and Pap stain, ×100, *Lower*).

Ancillary Studies

• Rearrangement of 8q11–13 is found in majority of cases and is diagnostically useful in doubtful cases.

Differential Diagnosis

• Myxoid liposarcoma,
• Lipoma NOS,
• Spindle cell lipoma,
• Hibernoma.

Atypical Lipomatous Tumor/Well-Differentiated Liposarcoma (Fig. 7.9)

ALT and WDL are synonyms because they have the same morphology, cytogenetic characteristics, and biological potential.

- They have a low malignant potential and are fatal only if not completely excised. The term WDL is retained only for tumors in the retroperitoneum and the mediastinum where complete resectability is usually questionable.
- ALT/WDL account for approximately 50% of all malignant adipocytic tumors. They occur in middle aged patients of both sexes in deep soft tissues of limbs, in retroperitoneum and in mediastinum.
- There are four histological variants of ALT/WDL: lipoma-like, sclerosing, inflammatory, and spindle cell. Tumors often contain two or even three different variants.

Cytomorphology of ALT/WDL

- Smears from ALT/WDL are usually not very cellular and unsatisfactory smears are much more frequent than in other types of liposarcoma.
- The lipoma-like variant is the most common. Smears usually contain tissue fragments with uniloculate adipocytes and stromal fragments with variable cellularity (Fig. 7.9).
- Univacuolated adipocytes can be mixed with many multivacuolated cells and/or small cells with oval nuclei. Some multivacuolated cells are similar to the ones described in lipomas while many of them have hyperchromatic nuclei (true lipoblasts) (Fig. 7.9).
- Majority of smears contain few scattered stromal cells with atypical nuclei which lie singly or in very small groups. The atypia varies from mild to severe in which case the hyperchromatic nuclei are large, round, oval, irregular, or lobulated (Fig. 7.9 upper, inset). Some cells are multinucleated and even arranged in a florette-like structure which is also characteristic for pleomorphic lipomas.[11,12] (Fig. 7.9)
- The background in ALT/WDL contains abundant free fat globules (Fig. 7.9) and sometimes a few histiocytes and fragments of striated muscle.

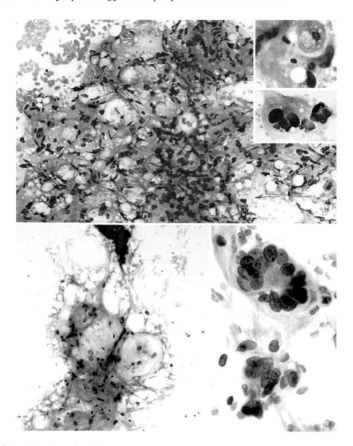

FIG. 7.9. **Atypical lipomatous tumor/well differentiated liposarcoma (ALT/WDL)**: *Upper*: A moderately cellular tissue fragment of ALT/WDL with many slightly atypical stromal cells and a few adipocytes. (DQ stain, ×200) Insert : A multivacuolated lipoblast, some endothelial cells, and a group of atypical cells. (DQ ×600). *Lower left*: A tissue fragment from ALT/WDL featuring atypical cells with oval nuclei and a fragment of striated muscle (red). (Pap stain, ×200). *Lower right*: a florette-like multinucleated cell. (Pap stain, ×600).

- In the sclerosing variant, the collagenous stroma predominates and areas containing the adipocytic component may not even be sampled. The same can be true for the inflammatory variant in which lymphocytic infiltrate can completely obscure the picture.

Ancillary Studies

- Demonstration of 12q14–15 amplification may be used in differentiating ALT/WDL from lipoma.

Differential Diagnosis

- Lipoma NOS when no atypical cells or stromal fragments are sampled
- Pleomorphic lipoma if lipoblasts are not found.

Adipocytic Tumors with Spindle Cells

Spindle Cell Lipoma (Fig. 7.10)

- Spindle cell lipoma belongs to the same category as pleomorphic lipoma. These two entities lie at the opposite ends of the spectrum and in between are tumors with features of both. Therefore some lipomas look completely bland while others have a certain degree of atypia.
- The typical location is in the back of the neck and shoulder area of elderly people, mostly men.
- These are benign lesions which rarely recur after local excision.

Cytomorphology of Spindle Cell Lipoma

- Spindle cell lipomas very often undergo extensive myxoid degeneration and so the majority of cases described in cytological literature had an appearance of a myxoid tumor.[13,14]
- The smears are not very cellular. Abundant myxoid material in the background contains tissue fragments with myxoid stroma, occasional capillary fragments and moderate number of cells (Fig. 7.10).
- Fragments with mature adipocyte are almost always present while tissue fragments with collagenous stroma are less common.
- Spindle cells predominate and range from uniform in some tumors to moderately pleomorphic in others.[15]
- Bland spindle cells have fine, fibrillary, elongated processes (Fig. 7.10).
- Atypical spindle cells have plump oval nuclei of variable size and are accompanied by rounded and polygonal cells with moderate amount of cytoplasm which can contain many small vacuoles (Fig. 7.10).

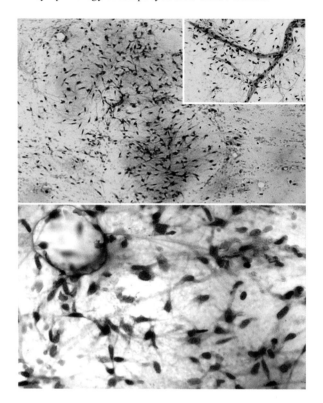

FIG. 7.10. **Spindle cell lipoma**: *Upper*: A tissue fragment with myxoid stroma, and moderate number of bland spindle cells. (DQ stain, ×100). Insert: a fragment with a prominent capillary network. *Lower*: Spindle cells with long cytoplasmic extensions. (DQ stain, ×600).

- An occasional multinucleated cell with a florette-like arrangement of nuclei may also be seen.
- The background contains dissociated tumor cells, rare cell groups without stroma, and most of the time also free fat globules and mastocytes.

Differential Diagnosis

- Pleomorphic lipoma,
- Myxoma,
- Myxoid neurofibroma,

- ALT/WDL-spindle cell variant,
- Myxoid liposarcoma,
- Low-grade myxofibrosarcoma.

Spindle Cell Variant of ALT/WDL (Fig. 7.11)

- This is only a morphological variety that does not have any clinical significance.

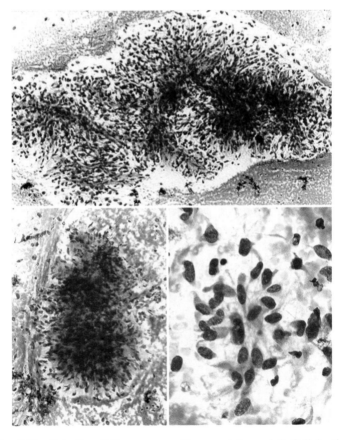

FIG. 7.11. **Spindle cell liposarcoma**: *Upper* and *Lower left*: Cellular tissue fragments containing capillaries; (DQ stain, ×100). *Lower right*: spindle cells with oval, hyperchromatic nuclei, slight pleomorphism and scant to moderate amounts of cytoplasm with long cytoplasmic extensions in some cells. (DQ stain, ×600).

Cytomorphology of Spindle Cell Variant of ALT/WDL

- Similar to the spindle cell lipoma, smears from spindle cell variant of ALT/WDL usually look like myxomatous tumors.
- Unlike lipomas they are highly cellular: there is dense cellularity in the tissue fragments and usually also among dissociated cells (Fig. 7.11).
- Nuclei are oval and hypochromatic, anisonucleosis is variable, cytoplasm scant (Fig. 7.11).
- Typical lipoblasts may not be present.

Differential Diagnosis

- Myxofibrosarcoma,
- Myxoid liposarcoma,
- Myxoid variant of Schwannoma.

Ancillary Studies

- MDM2 and CDK4 (both together are sensitive and specific)
- S100 (adipocytes), and CD34 (some spindle cells).
- Ring or giant marker/rod chromosomes derived from 12q13-15 in almost all cases.
- MDM2 and CDK4 by FISH or real time PCR can separate from other sarcomas.

Myxoid Adipocytic Tumors

Myxoid Liposarcoma (Figs. 7.12 and 7.13)

- This is the second largest group of liposarcomas affecting one-third of all liposarcoma patients.
- Most common locations are deep tissues of the extremities especially the thigh.
- 40- and 50-year-old patients are most commonly affected.
- Myxoid liposarcoma recurs locally and has a unique pattern of metastasizing to the opposite extremity, to the retroperitoneum, axilla, and spine.
- High-grade tumors have cellular areas with round cell morphology, the so-called round cell liposarcoma which used to be considered a separate entity (Fig. 7.13).

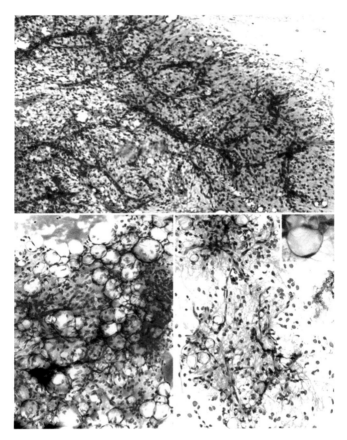

FIG. 7.12. **Myxoid liposarcoma**: Tissue fragments are highly cellular and usually contain extensive capillary networks; (DQ stain, ×200). The stroma is Myxoid and a few signet ring lipoblasts are seen (Insert).

Cytomorphology of Myxoid Liposarcoma

- Smears from myxoid liposarcomas have abundant myxoid material in the background and various numbers of tissue fragments and dissociated cells.
- Tissue fragments are composed of myxoid stroma containing an extensive vascular pattern and nonlipogenic mesenchymal

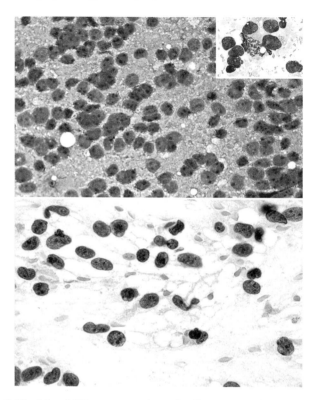

FIG. 7.13. **Myxoid liposarcoma (round cell component)**: Naked nuclei can predominate the smear; mitotic figures are common. (DQ stain, ×400, *Upper*: Pap stain, ×600 *Lower*).

cells.[16,17] The cellularity of tissue fragments ranges from low to high (Fig. 7.12).

- Some fragments also contain many adipocytes and very often lipoblasts with multivacuolated or monovacuolated cytoplasm (signet ring lipoblasts).
- Nonlipogenic cells have oval or plump nuclei which can be uni-morphous or show slight to moderate polymorphism. Cytoplasm can have long fibrillary processes or it is scant and rounded (Figs. 7.12 and 7.13).

Ancillary Studies

- 90% of myxoid liposarcomas, including those with round cell areas, have translocation[12–16](q13;p11) which can be demonstrated by FISH in morphologically doubtful cases.

Differential Diagnosis

- Spindle cell lipoma,
- Spindle cell variant of ALT/WDL,
- Lipoblastoma,
- Myxofibrosarcoma.

Myxomatous Variants of Other Adipocytic Tumors

Myxomatous degeneration of stroma is very common in most adipocytic tumors except in pure lipomas where it is rare. Therefore smears from various adipocytic tumors can contain myxomatous material in the background and in tissue fragments. Sometimes only scant fragments are seen; however, very often myxomatous stroma is abundant.

Round Cell Adipocytic Tumors

Round Cell Liposarcoma

- Round cell liposarcoma used to be classified as a separate entity. Since it shares the same karyotype with the myxoid liposarcoma it is now considered only as a variant of the myxoid liposarcoma.
- In histological sections there is gradual transition from myxoid to the round cell areas. Cytological smears may contain only the round cell variant of liposarcoma or fragments of both types.
- The round cell component is a high-grade tumor and it foretells a poor prognosis if there are more than 25% round cell areas.[18]

Cytomorphology of Round Cell Liposarcoma

- Smears from the round cell areas are highly cellular and composed predominantly of dissociated cells and naked nuclei.

- Tissue fragments may be present.
- Cells are round with high nuclear/cytoplasmic ratios, hyper-chromasia, and multiple small nucleoli. The degree of aniso-nucleosis varies from monomorphous to moderate in various cases.
- Some authors mention that cytoplasm of some round cell liposa-rcoma cells contains many small vacuoles; however, in our opin-ion these cells come from the myxoid areas rather than from the round cell areas of the tumor.[2]
- Typical lipoblasts are rare, mitotic figures are frequent.
- Background is granular.

Ancillary Studies

- Immunocytochemical demonstration of S100 protein is useful in the differential diagnosis with other morphologically similar tumors; however, all cases are not positive.

Pleomorphic Adipocytic Tumors

Pleomorphic Lipoma (Fig. 7.14)

- As already mentioned in the section on spindle cell adipocytic tumors, pleomorphic lipoma belongs to the same category with spindle cell lipoma. Clinical and genetic characteristics are the same in both.

Cytomorphology of Pleomorphic Lipoma

- In adequate samples, smears should contain fragments of mature adipocytes and dissociated cells which range from spindle to round and polygonal with various amounts of ill-defined cyto-plasm (Fig. 7.14).
- There is pronounced anisonucleosis with bi- and multinucleated cells, some with the florette appearance. Individual nuclei are hyperchromatic.
- As in spindle cell lipomas, there can be myxoid material in the background (Fig. 7.14).

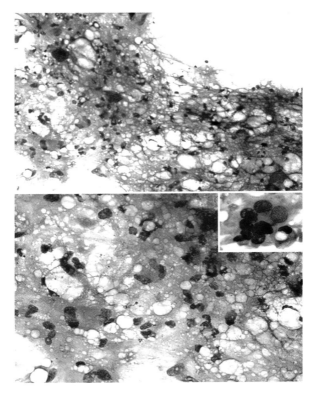

Fig. 7.14. **Pleomorphic lipoma**: Myxoid stroma contains many free fat droplets, a few adipocytes and a polymorphous cell population with oval or round nuclei, moderate or abundant cytoplasm, pronounced aniso-nucleosis. (DQ stain, ×200 (*Upper*); x 400 (*Lower*); Insert: A multinucle-ated, rosette-like cell.

- The separation of pleomorphic lipoma from spindle cell lipoma may not always be possible and a clear distinction from ALT/ WDL is questionable in cytology.
- As López-Ríos pointed out, many pitfalls have been reported and the diagnosis should be rendered only when there is excel-lent clinical and cytological correlation.[19]

Differential Diagnosis

- Spindle cell lipoma,
- ALT/WDL, carcinoma.

Pleomorphic Liposarcoma (Fig. 7.15)

- Pleomorphic liposarcoma is the least common variant of liposarcomas.

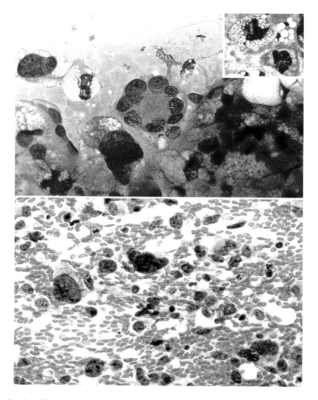

FIG. 7.15. **Pleomorphic liposarcoma**: *Upper*: A tissue fragment with many multivacuolated lipoblasts and multinucleated pleomorphic tumor cells, (DQ stain, ×600). *Lower*: A mixed population of small and large sarcoma cells. (Pap stain, ×400).

- It arises in elderly patients, predominately in the limbs and has no sex predilection.
- Pleomorphic liposarcoma is a high-grade sarcoma, which metastasizes most often to the lungs. Recurrence rate and mortality rate are around 50% and time between diagnosis and death is shorter than in other liposarcomas or others pleomorphic sarcomas.

Cytomorphology of Pleomorphic Liposarcoma

- There is great variability in the morphological picture seen in FNA samples.
- Cell clusters and dissociated cells can be numerous. In an alternative picture, dissociated cells predominate (Fig. 7.15).
- Cell morphology is also highly variable: primitive, small mesenchymal cells admixed with large pleomorphic ones; predominance of pleomorphic spindle cells or epithelioid cells.[20] (Fig. 7.15)
- Giant tumor cells are common, often multinucleated but may not be numerous (Fig. 7.15).
- Number of multivacuolated lipoblasts is variable.
- Background can contain myxoid material (Fig. 7.15), necrotic debris, inflammatory cells, and free fat globules.

Ancillary Studies

- S-100 protein, which is a marker for adipocytic tumors, is positive in approximately half of the pleomorphic liposarcoma cases.
- Cytogenetic analysis is not very helpful in the differential diagnosis because there is no consistent chromosomal aberration.

Differential Diagnosis

- All other pleomorphic sarcomas,
- Myxofibrosarcoma,
- Metastatic poorly differentiated carcinoma.

Dedifferentiated Liposarcoma (Fig. 7.16)

- A form of liposarcoma composed of areas of ALT/WDL and areas of nonlipogenic sarcoma (the dedifferentiated component).

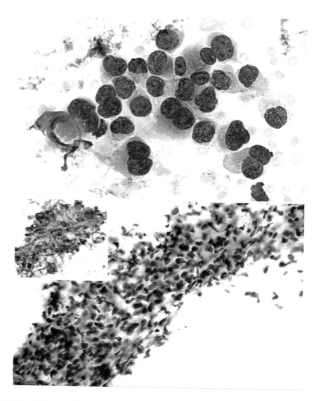

FIG. 7.16. *Upper*: Dedifferentiated liposarcoma with focal rhabdomyosarcomatous features. (DQ stain, ×600) *Lower*: a high grade spindle cell sarcoma; (Pap stain, ×400) Insert: positive reaction for desmin.

- It is most often seen in the retroperitoneum.
- Radiological pictures show a lipomatous and a nonlipomatous component.
- Dedifferentiated liposarcoma behaves less aggressively than other pleomorphic sarcomas.
- The dedifferentiated component is most commonly a high-grade sarcoma (MFH-like or myxofibrosarcoma).
- A low-grade dedifferentiated component is usually a spindle cell one with mild atypia.

- Heterologous dedifferentiated component can be rhabdomyosarcoma (Fig. 7.16), osteosarcoma, and chondrosarcoma.

Cytomorphology of Dedifferentiated Liposarcoma

- Reliable diagnosis from FNA smears is seldom possible because rarely both components are sampled even if multiple passes are made.
- The cytological diagnosis is therefore either ALT/WDL or a nonlipogenic sarcoma, depending on the area sampled.
- There is no characteristic picture in FNA samples. Smears can be highly cellular containing groups and dissociated cells with obvious malignant features, spindle-shaped cells or mixed spindle and round cells (Fig. 7.16).
- An alternative picture features few cells with mild atypia.[7–16]
- There is often myxoid material in the background.
- The presence of heterologous sarcoma cells from a retroperitoneal tumor may help in suggesting the correct diagnosis since rhabdomyosarcoma, osteosarcoma, and chondrosarcomas are rare or nonexistent in this location.

Pitfalls in Adipocytic Tumors

- Degenerative changes in lipoma produce atypia and vacuolated macrophages may simulate lipoblasts, creating an appearance similar to ALT/WDL.[21]
- FNA samples from ALT/WDL can simulate a lipoma when representative atypical cells and/or lipoblasts are not present.
- Pleomorphic lipoma closely mimics ALT/WDL and clear separation of the two entities is questionable in cytology.
- Spindle cell lipoma should not be mistaken for a myxoid liposarcoma or a low-grade myxofibrosarcoma.
- Lipoblastoma is morphologically similar to myxoid liposarcoma; the young age of the patient is helpful in making the right diagnosis.
- Chondroid lipoma resembles myxoid liposarcoma; chondroid material is the clue to the right diagnosis.
- Myxoid liposarcoma may not contain pronounced atypia or many lipoblasts and can be mistaken for a spindle cell lipoma or a myxoma.

- Round cell liposarcoma cannot be distinguished from lymphoma or from other round cell neoplasms without the aid of immuno-cytochemistry.
- Pleomorphic liposarcoma cannot be separated from other pleomorphic sarcomas solely on the basis of morphology. Even more important is its identity from a metastatic carcinoma.
- Dedifferentiated liposarcoma contains spindle or pleomorphic cells of nonadipocytic lineage and therefore can seldom be diagnosed correctly in cytology since immunocytochemistry is misleading in such cases.

References

1. Fletcher CDM, Uni KK, Mertens F, eds. *World Health Organization Classification of tumors. Pathology and Genetics. Tumors of Soft Tissue and Bone*. Lyon: IARC Press; 2002:19–46.
2. Layfield LJ. Lipomatous neoplasms. In: *Cytopathology of bone and soft tissue tumors* Layfield LJ (ed); Oxford University Press, Inc. New York 2002; p 71–74.
3. Akerman M, Domansky HA. Adipocytic tumors. In: Orell SR, Karger S, AG Basel, eds. *Monographs in Clinical Cytology, the Cytology of Soft Tissue Tumors, vol. 16*. 2003:17–19.
4. Gisselsson D, Domanski HA, Höglund M. Unique cytological features and chromosome aberrations in chondroid lipoma. A case report based on fine-needle aspiration cytology, histopathology electron microscopy, chromosome banding, and molecular cytogenetics. *Am J Surg Pathol*. 1999;23:1300–1304.
5. Hashimoto CH, Cobb CJ. Cytodiagnosis of hibernoma: a case report. *Diagn Cytopathol*. 1987;3:326–329.
6. Kloboves Prevodnik V, Us Krašovec M, Gale N, Lamovec J. Cytological features of lipoblastoma: a report of three cases. *Diagn Cytopathol*. 2005;33:195–200.
7. Pollono DG, Tomarchio S, Drut R. Retroperitoneal and deep-seated lipoblastoma: diagnosis by CT scan and fine-needle aspiration biopsy. *Diagn Cytopathol*. 1999;20:295–297.
8. Leon ME, Deschler D, Wu SS, Galindo LM. Fine needle aspiration diagnosis of lipoblastoma of the parotid region. A case report. *Acta Cytol*. 2002;46:395–404.
9. Talwar MB, Misra K, Marya SKS, Dev G. Fine needle aspiration cytology of a lipoblastoma. *Acta Cytol*. 1990;34:855–857.

2. Soft tissue mass resection margin: With clear orientation by the surgeon, the exterior is inked and serially cross-sectioned. A careful gross examination of the exterior and interior of the tumor is conducted to identify areas suspicious for margin involvement. Frozen section biopsies of suspicious areas are performed judiciously. If margins are clear, the specimen can then be processed for permanent section and definitive evaluation. For the evaluation of soft tissue margins, we don't believe that cytology plays any practical role.

3. Biopsy of bone and soft tissue lesions for intraoperative diagnosis: Bone or soft tissue mass biopsy is usually necessary for first time diagnosis and when tissue confirmation is essential before initiation of therapy. Realistic expectations for intraoperative pathologic diagnosis include the following:

   (a) Determining whether a lesion is benign or malignant. If malignant, further determinations are needed to ascertain lymphoma/plasmacytoma, metastatic disease, or mesenchymal primary.
   (b) Being aware that subtyping of a tumor is not always possible. It is important to obtain representative tissue samples, establish a differential diagnosis, and appropriately triage the tissue to facilitate a definitive diagnosis on permanent section.

Cytological Preparations

1. Touch imprint: This is done by gently touching the surface of the specimen without disturbing the integrity of the core or resection specimen. The imprint slide is air-dried and stained with the Diff-Quik (DQ) method. Touch imprints can screen the cellularity and quality of a specimen and aid in selection of appropriate core for frozen section (Fig. 8.2). If cytology reveals a hypocellular specimen, additional tissue can be requested. For serially sectioned larger masses, this method can screen the entire tumor surface and provide added valuable information to frozen section alone. Additional alcohol-fixed slides can be prepared for Papanicolaou (PAP) stain.

2. Scrape smear: This is done by using one end of a glass slide to gently scrape the surface of the lesion and to make a thin-layer smear, which is then air-dried and DQ stained. This method generates

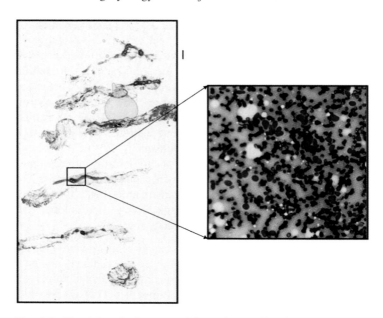

FIG. 8.2. Touch imprint is prepared from six core biopsies. Core *number 4* from the top is cellular and chosen for frozen section to facilitate the intraoperative diagnosis, DQ, x1 (*left*), and DQ, x400 (*right*).

more cellular slides and is useful in evaluating hypocellular lesions and in collecting cellular specimens for ancillary study.

These cytological preparations are done before frozen section. Additional air-dried and unstained slides from both methods can be made for ancillary studies. We cannot emphasize enough that the best opportunity to preserve tissue for ancillary studies is at fresh tissue evaluation and that formalin-fixed tissues provide less optimal samples for ancillary studies. Fresh tissue can be collected for flow cytometry (in RPMI), karyotyping (in RPMI), electron microscopy (in 3% glutaraldehyde), FISH (unstained touch imprints, smears, and cytospin), and molecular studies (in RNA preservative). In our experience, it is critical to reserve tissue for ancillary studies and subsequent confirmation.

Case Illustrations of the Most Commonly Encountered Clinical Scenario in Which Cytology Enhances the Intraoperative Diagnosis of Sarcoma

1. *Frozen section reveals a poorly differentiated malignancy of round cells (Fig. 8.3)*

Key points: The differential diagnosis includes metastatic carcinoma or melanoma, lymphoma or plasmacytoma, and sarcoma. Clinical history is important in separating these tumors, but this can be confusing when the patient does not have known history of malignancy or has multiple different prior tumors. However, the immediate surgical management warrants identification of for sarcoma vs. nonsarcoma. In this situation, a touch imprint of the lesion can help significantly in the diagnosis of lymphoma (Fig. 8.4), plasmacytoma (Fig. 8.5), or carcinoma (Fig. 8.6). If a hematopoietic malignancy is favored, fresh tissue can be submitted for flow cytometry analysis. Additional unstained touch imprint slides can be prepared for gene rearrangement study. If a carcinoma is favored, touch imprint slides can be used for rapid cytokeratin stain for confirmation, similar to that done for sentinel

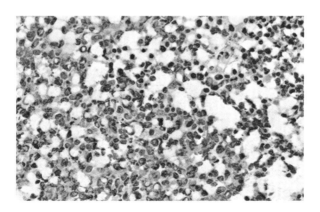

FIG. 8.3. Frozen section slides (H&E, ×400) reveal a poorly differentiated malignancy of round cells with frozen artifact. No definitive pattern or matrix is identified.

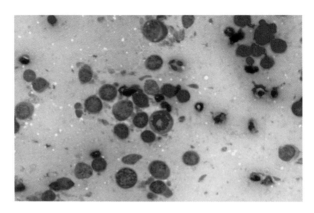

FIG. 8.4. Touch imprint (DQ, ×600) reveals highly malignant cells with frequent mitosis and abundant lymphoglandular bodies. Consequent flow cytometry confirms that this is a diffuse large B-cell lymphoma. Cytology slides can be further used for gene rearrangement study.

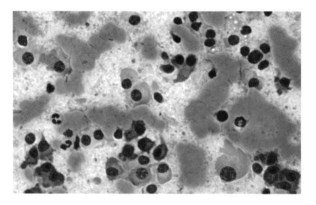

FIG. 8.5. Touch imprint (DQ, ×600) reveals plasmacytoid cells with clock-faced nuclei and binucleation. Consequent flow cytometry also confirms it as plasmacytoma.

lymph node of breast cancer (Fig. 8.7). If a sarcoma is favored (Fig. 8.8), fresh tissue can be submitted for cytogenetic karyo-typing. Additional unstained cytology slides can be prepared for FISH study (Fig. 8.8, inset), to facilitate a future definitive diagnosis. Sarcomas with round cell cytomorphology include Ewing

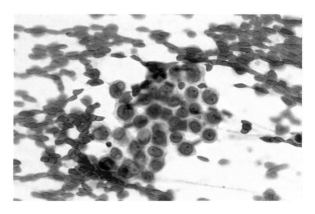

FIG. 8.6. Intracytoplasmic lumen is evident on touch imprint cytology (PAP, ×400), consistent with a metastatic adenocarcinoma.

FIG. 8.7. A case of right humerus lesion with a history of lobular carcinoma of the breast and melanoma, the tumor cells are dyshesive and plasmacytoid. No melanin pigment is identified. Rapid cytokeratin stain (CK, ×600) done on touch imprint slides with appropriate controls reveals numerous cytokeratin-positive cells and confirms the diagnosis of a metastatic carcinoma, compatible with history of breast cancer.

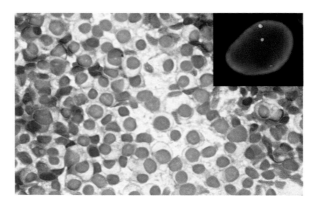

FIG. 8.8. Touch imprint cytology (DQ, ×600) reveals dispersed, small, *blue round cells* without lymphoglandular bodies, dimorphic "light" and "dark" cells, and vacuolated cytoplasm, suggestive of Ewing sarcoma/ PNET. *Insert*: Cytology slides were submitted for FISH study, which is useful for sarcomas with known translocations. With this method, it takes less time to confirm a diagnosis than karyotyping (see Tables 8.1 and 9.1). In this case, Ewing sarcoma is confirmed by identifying t(11;22) (q24;q12) in interphase nuclei. A representative nucleus is shown in insert (FISH, ×1000).

TABLE 8.1. Confirmation of diagnosis via karyotyping vs. FISH.

	Karyotype	FISH
Tissue	Fresh, grown for metaphase spread	Cytology slides, FFPE[a] slides
Cell growth	Yes	No
Detection	Global cytogenetic defect (numerical and structural)	Defined translocation
Time	More than 2 weeks	Overnight

[a]Formalin fixed paraffin embedded

sarcoma/PNET, desmoplastic small round cell tumor, rhabdomyosarcoma, and extraskeletal myxoid chondrosarcoma.

2. *Frozen section reveals a myxoid or fatty lesion*
Key points: The differential diagnosis includes myxomas, liposarcoma (especially myxoid liposarcoma), chordoma, myxoid chondrosarcoma, other myxoid spindle/pleomorphic cell sarcoma, and

mucinous carcinoma. The diagnosis of these tumors can be greatly enhanced by adjunct cytology (Figs. 8.9–8.13). When a definitive diagnosis is not possible intraoperatively, the advantage of adjunct cytology imprint of the specimen is the ability to evaluate whether the tissue is cellular or sufficient enough for a diagnostic work-up. If not, additional tissue can be requested. If the tissue is sufficient, that is, a cellular specimen with large amounts of atypical cells, fresh tissue should be submitted for cytogenetic karyotyping and additional unstained cytology slides should be prepared for FISH study which can confirm myxoid liposarcoma and extraskeletal myxoid chondrosarcoma.

3. *Frozen section reveals a spindle cell lesion*
Key points: This differential diagnosis is broad ranging, from non-neoplastic to neoplastic, benign to malignant. Nodular fasciitis, fibromatosis (desmoids tumor), leiomyoma, leiomyosarcoma, benign peripheral nerve sheath tumor, malignant nerve sheath tumor, gastrointestinal tumor, various fibroblastic/myofibroblastic and fibrohistiocytic tumors, malignant melanoma, and spindle cell carcinoma are among this long list of differential diagnoses. Cytology can help to confirm whether it is mesenchymal; the relative grade of the tumor, therefore, offers guidance to subsequent management (Figs. 8.14 and 8.15).

4. *Frozen section reveals a chondroid lesion*
Key points: The differential diagnosis of this group includes chondroma, chondrosarcoma, and others. A definitive diagnosis relies on radiological features and the histological examination of the entire lesion. Intraoperative consultation is limited to providing information regarding the tissue adequacy and to rule out a high-grade sarcoma (Fig. 8.16).

5. *Frozen section reveals a giant cell rich lesion*
Key points: The differential diagnosis includes giant cell tumor of bone, giant cell tumor of tendon sheath, chondroblastoma, giant cell reparative granuloma, and sarcoma with giant cells. Intraoperative consultation is limited to providing information regarding the tissue adequacy, confirm it is a giant cell rich lesion, and to rule out a high-grade sarcoma (Fig. 8.17), which requires different immediate surgical management.

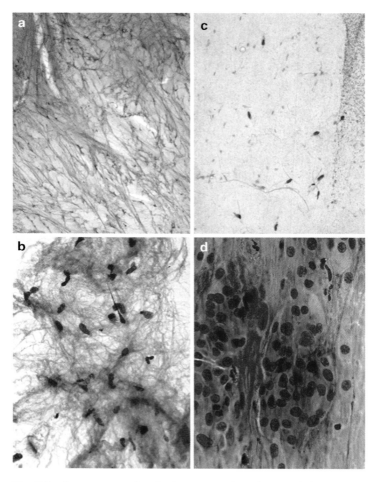

FIG. 8.9. Scrape smear of multiple cross-section of a myxoid lesion, with a homogenous cut surface, reveals a hypocellular smear with (**a**) (DQ, ×100) abundant myxoid matrix and (**b**) (DQ, ×200) bland spindle cells, which is diagnostic for myxoma. Another myxoid lesion shows increased cellularity but still bland cells (**c**) (DQ, ×400), seen in intramuscular myxoma or cellular myxoma. A myxoid lesion with pleomorphic cells and frequent mitosis is indicative of a high-grade sarcoma with myxoid changes (**d**) (DQ, ×600), a situation showing that ancillary study is warranted for further classification.

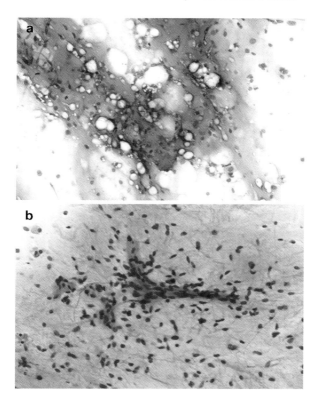

Fig. 8.10. A grossly fatty and myxoid lesion reveals on scrape smear (**a**) (DQ, ×200) an abundant myxoid matrix with lipoblasts and (**b**) (DQ, ×400) with delicate vessels, suggestive of a myxoid liposarcoma. Fresh tissue for karyotyping or unstained smears for FISH should be submitted for confirmation.

In this chapter, we presented a practical, algorithmic approach to the intraoperative diagnosis of sarcoma with adjunct cytology. We hope that this approach can be applied to the daily practice of surgical pathology of bone and soft tissue lesions and aid the diagnosis and subsequent management.

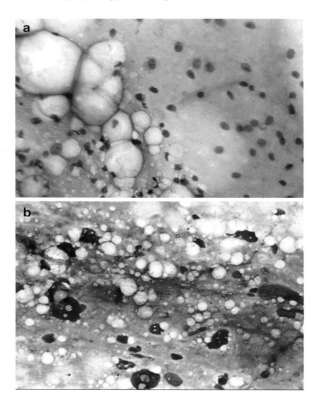

FIG. 8.11. Scrape smear from a grossly large, fatty, and heterogeneous tumor showing fatty background with large hyperchromatic cells, suggestive of a liposarcoma (**a**) (DQ, ×400) with areas of high-grade dedifferentiation (**b**) (DQ, ×400).

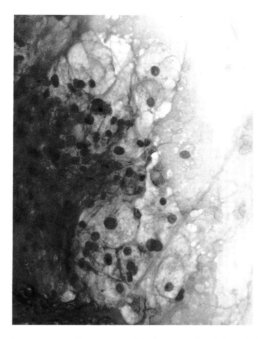

Fig. 8.12. Scrape smear from a sacral lesion reveals (DQ, ×400) fibrillary myxoid matrix and cohesive clusters and cords of large cells. The cytoplasm is abundant with conspicuous cytoplasmic vacuoles. Physaliphorous cells are seen. The cytological differential diagnosis includes chordoma, myxopapillary ependymoma, extraskelatal myxoid chondrosarcoma, and mucinous adenocarcinoma. However, the location of this lesion is consistent with a chordoma.

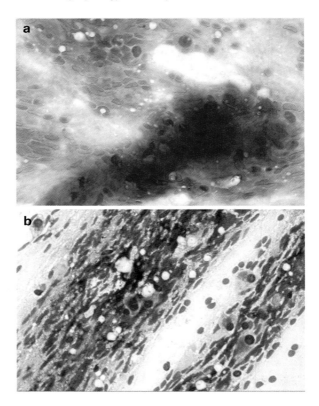

FIG. 8.13. Scrape smear reveals (**a**) (DQ, ×400) bright magenta fibrillary stroma with (**b**) (DQ, ×400) bland and uniform cells, suggestive of extraskeletal myxoid chondrosaroma. When this diagnosis is one of the differential diagnoses during intraopeative pathologic consultation, fresh tissue needs to be submitted for karyotyping and unstained cytology slides needs to be prepared. If confirmation of extraskeletal myxoid chondrosarcoma is needed, they can be submitted for FISH testing.

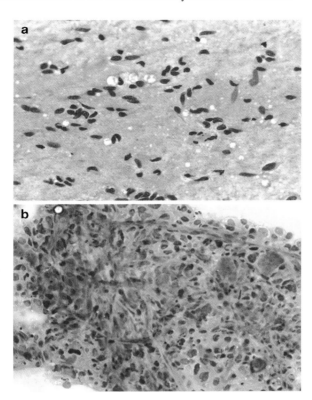

FIG. 8.14. Shown is a spindle cell lesion with hypercellularity and collagenous/myxoid background and mild nuclear pleomorphism (**a**) (DQ, ×400). The cytomorphology suggests a benign to low-grade mesenchymal neoplasm. Ancillary studies are warranted for further classification. This case was a spindle cell sarcoma, NOS, low grade with focal intermediate area. Also shown is a very cellular spindle cell lesion with obvious nuclear pleomorphism (**b**) (DQ, ×200). The cytomorphology suggests a malignant mesenchymal tumor. Ancillary studies are warranted for further classification. This case was a high-grade leiomyosarcoma.

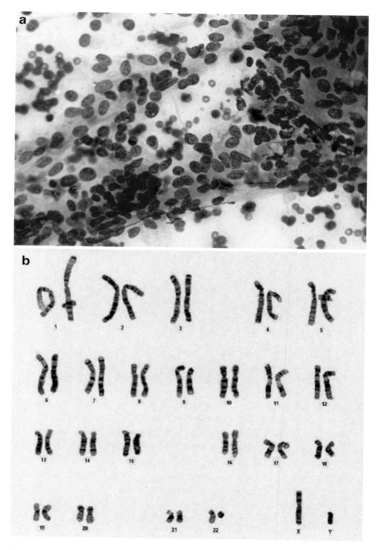

FIG. 8.15 Shown is a hypercellular spindle cell tumor with relative monotonous and overlapping nuclei, suggestive of a synovial sarcoma (**a**) (DQ, ×400). Karyotyping confirms the diagnosis by identifying the characteristic t(x;18) translocation (**b**).

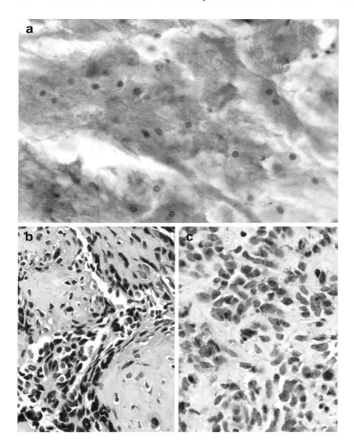

FIG. 8.16.   Shown is a chondroid lesion with bland round cells with eosinophilic cells, consistent with a benign or low-grade cartilaginous lesion (**a**) (DQ, ×400). Also shown is a biphasic malignant chondroid lesion with small round to oval cells consistent with a mesenchymal chondrosarcoma (**b**) (H&E, ×600); the cellular component was better captured by scrape smear with dense matrix (**c**) (DQ, ×600).

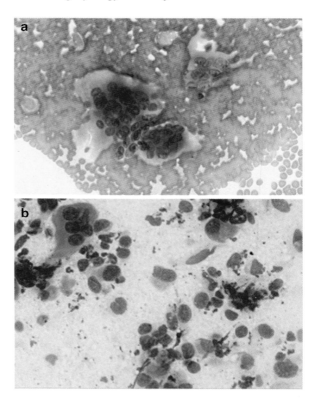

FIG. 8.17. Touch imprint reveals (**a**) (DQ, ×600) a giant cell rich lesion with no evidence of malignancy and (**b**) (QD, ×600) a high-grade osteosarcoma with therapy effect.

References

1. Ashford RU, McCarthy SW, Scolyer RA, et al. Surgical biopsy with intra-operative frozen section. An accurate and cost-effective method for diagnosis of musculoskeletal sarcomas. *J Bone Joint Surg Br.* 2006;88:1207–1211.
2. Domanski HA, Akerman M, Carlen B, et al. Core-needle biopsy performed by cytopathologist: a technique to complement fine-needle aspiration of soft tissue and bone lesions. *Cancer.* 2005;105:229–239.
3. Bui MM, Smith P, Agresta SV, Cheong D, Letson GD. Practical issues of intraoperative frozen section diagnosis of bone and soft tissue lesions. *Cancer Control.* 2008;15(1):7–12.

9
Ancillary Studies in FNAC of Soft Tissue and Bone Lesions

Marilyn M. Bui[1] and Walid E. Khalbuss[2]

[1] Moffitt Cancer Center, Tampa, FL, USA

[2] University of Pittsburgh Medical Center, UPMC-Shadyside, POB2, Suite 201 Cytology, 5150 Centre Avenue, Pittsburgh, PA 15232, USA

Fine needle aspiration biopsy is useful in the diagnosis of bone and soft tissue tumors, especially for superficial primary sarcomas and metastatic or recurrent disease. The rinse of the biopsy needle often generates an adequate tissue for cell block preparation, which is a valuable source of specimen for ancillary studies. Ancillary studies generally include immunocytochemistry (IHC), cytogenetic karyotyping, flow cytometry, electron microscopy (EM), fluorescence in situ hybridization (FISH), reverse transcriptase polymerase chain reaction (RT-PCR), and mutational analysis. Karyotyping (will detect structural and numerical chromosomal abnormality when sarcoma is suspected, Table 9.1) and flow cytometry (will detect the clonality when lymphoma is suspected) require fresh tumor sample.

In recent years, IHC has become the most commonly or routinely used method in identifying the lineage and differentiation of mesenchymal tumors because of its relative ease of use and interpretation. Meanwhile, the use of EM has declined but reserves a role for poorly differentiated mesenchymal tumors that are negative or nonspecific for antigenic expression. IHC is superior in diagnosis of smooth muscle tumors, small round cell tumors, sarcomas with epithelioid morphology, and most synovial sarcomas[1]; while EM is particularly valuable for peripheral nerve sheath tumors, marker-negative synovial sarcomas, pleomorphic

W.E. Khalbuss and A.V. Parwani, *Cytopathology of Soft Tissue and Bone Lesions*, Essentials in Cytopathology 9, DOI 10.1007/978-1-4419-6499-1_9, © Springer Science+Business Media, LLC 2011

TABLE 9.1. Most common cytogenetic alterations in bone and soft tissue sarcomas.

Tumor	Cytogenetic alterations	Frequency (%)
Alveolar soft part sarcoma	t(x:17)(p11;q25)	90
Clear cell sarcoma	t(11;22)(q13;q12)	75
Dermatofibrosarcoma protuberans	Chromosome 17 and 22 ring forms	80
	t(17;22)(q22;q13)	10
Desmoplastic small round cell tumor	t(11;22)(p13;q12)	75
Ewing sarcoma/primitive neutoectodermal tumor	t(11;22)(q24;q12)	80
	t(21;22)(q12;q12)	5
	t(2;22)(q33;q12)	<5
	t(7;22)(p22;q12)	<5
	t(17;22)(q12;q12)	<5
	inv.(22)(q12;q12)	<5
Extraskeletal myxoid chondrosarcoma	t(9;22)(q22;q12)	80
	t(9;17)(q22;q11)	10
	t(9;15)(q22;q12)	10
Liposarcoma, well differentiated	Chromosome 12 (giant marker chromosomes and/or ring chromosomes)	80
Liposarcoma, myxoid/round cell	t(12;16)(q13;p11)	80
	t(12;22)(q13;q12)	5
Low-grade fibromyxoid sarcoma	t(7;16)(9q32-34;q11)	50
Rhabdomyosarcoma, alveolar	t(2;13)(q35;q14)	80
	t(1;3)(p36;q14)	20
Rhabdomyosarcoma, embryonal	Trisomies 2q, 8 and 20	75
	Loss of heterozygosity at 11p15	75
Schwannoma	Deletion of 22q	80
Synovial sarcoma	t(x;18)(p11;q11)	90

sarcomas, mesotheliomas, alveloar soft part sarcoma, and clear cell sarcoma.[1–3] This chapter will focus on the role of immunocytochemical studies and other molecular studies such as FISH, RT-PCR, and mutational analysis in the diagnosis of sarcomas.

According to the cytomorphology, mesenchymal tumors can be arbitrarily divided into the following groups: spindle cell, round cell, epithelioid cell, lipoid cell, and pleomorphic cell morphology. Each group has certain common differential diagnoses. A panel of immunocytochemical markers can then be used to further differentiate the tumor. In conjunction with clinical and radiological information, a definitive diagnosis can be reached.

Spindle Cell Malignancy

Differential diagnosis includes spindle cell melanoma, spindle cell carcinoma, and spindle cell sarcoma (Table 9.2). Cytokeratin (CK) is a commonly used marker to rule out carcinoma; however, focal CK expression can be seen in sarcomas. Synovial sarcoma, epithelioid sarcoma (ES), epithelioid angiosarcoma, and Ewing sarcoma frequently demonstrate CK expression.[4,5] CK and epithelial membrane antigen (EMA) are positive in both spindle cell carcinoma and synovial sarcoma. However, CD99 (MIC2) and BCL-2 are mostly positive in synovial sarcoma. Most spindle cell melanomas express S-100 protein and it may be the only positive makers among other melanocytic markers such as HMB-45 (50% expression), Melan-A and Tyrosinase. Comparing spindle cell melanoma to peripheral nerve sheath tumor, the S-100 expression is usually focal in the latter. H-Caldesmon is expressed in most smooth muscle tumors, while desmin is usually positive in 50% of extrauterine leiomyosarcomas (Fig. 9.1). Benign neural tumor is usually strongly and diffusely positive for S-100 (Fig. 9.2). Gastrointestinal stromal tumor (GIST) is most often positive for CD 117 and CD34. Of note, vimentin has no role in separating the above tumors because of lack of specificity.

For synovial sarcoma (SS), the t (x;18) translocation is the hallmark cytogenetic abnormality seen in greater than 90% of tumors (Fig. 9.3). FISH technique (Fig. 9.3) or RT-PCR can be used to detect tumor RNA from cell block material for SYT-SSX transcripts. Molecular testing is not required to make a definitive diagnosis of SS, if clinical, morphological and immunocytological findings support the diagnosis. However, molecular testing has proven very helpful in cases when SS is one of the differential diagnoses and warrants further confirmation.[6] Prognostically, patients with the SYT/SSX1 fusion gene product have a poor clinical outcome.[7–9] Other common sarcoma specific fusion transcripts detected by RT-PCR are listed in Table 9.3. In addition, RT-PCR is also ideal in detecting the KIT and PDGFR gene mutation in

TABLE 9.2. Differentiating immunostain pattern of spindle cell malignancy.

	CK	EMA	S-100	HMB-45	Desmin	H-Caldesmon	CD99 (MIC 2)	CD117 (C-KIT)
Spindle cell melanoma	–	–	+ Diffuse	±	–	–	–	–
Spindle cell carcinoma	+	+	–	–	–	–	–	–
Synovial sarcoma	+	+	–/+	–	–	–	+	–
Malignant nerve sheath tumor	–	–	+ Focal	–	–	–	–	–
Leiomyosarcoma	–	–	–	–	±	+	–	–
GIST	–	–	–	–	–	–	–	+

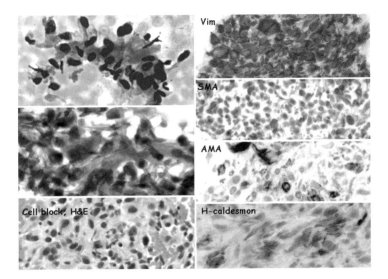

FIG. 9.1. Ancillary studies in metastatic leiomyosarcoma. A 53-year-old women with an iliac bone destructive lesion. She has history of hysterectomy for leiomyosarcoma 3 years prior. CT-guided FNA of iliac lesion (DQ- and Pap-stained smears, ×600 magnification, cell block H&E, ×400, and immunostain study on cell block, *right*). The tumor was positive for vimentin, actin, AMA, and H-Caldesmon. Metastatic leiomyosarcoma was confirmed and clinically it was uterine primary.

GIST, especially when there is no immunocytologically evidence of CD117 or CD34 expression, but clinically strong suspicion for GIST.[10]

Round Cell Malignancy

Differential diagnosis includes small cell carcinoma, lymphoma, seminoma, Ewing/PNET, desmoplastic small round cell tumor (DSRCT), and rhabdomyosarcoma (Table 9.4). CK expression is seen in most carcinomas. Small cell carcinoma is also reactive to synaptophysin, chromogranin, CD56, and NSE. CD45 (leukocyte common antigen) is a sensitive and specific lymphoma marker,

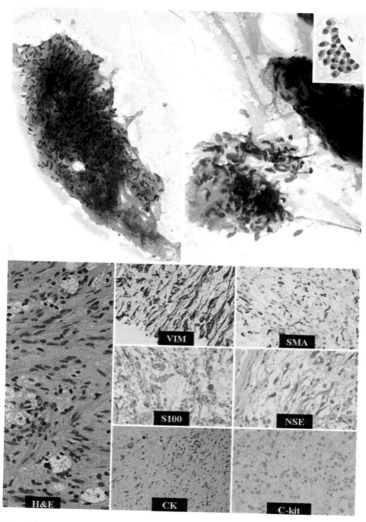

Fig. 9.2. Ancillary study in neurogenic tumor. This is FNA of a neck soft tissue mass with history of a slow-growing painful mass. The DQ stain reveals a spindle mesenchymal lesion with minimal cytological atypia (*left* and *right upper*, x200 & 400 respectively). The cell block shows a relatively hypocellular spindle cell tumor with no significant cytological atypia (H&E, x200). Numerous form cells are noted. A panel of immunostains reveals the tumor cells are positive for vimentin and S-100, but negative for SMA, NSE, CK, and C-KIT, supporting the diagnosis of benign neurogenic tumor consistent with neurofibroma or schwannoma.

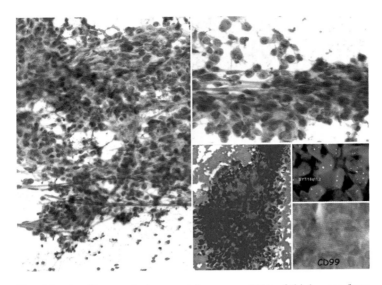

Fig. 9.3. Ancillary study in synovial sarcoma. FNA of thigh mass from a 69-year-old female (Pap stained, x200 & x400 and DQ-stained smears x100 and CD99 immunostain and FISH study). The tumor is immunoreactive for CD99. The FISH study is positive for t(x;18)(p11;q11) confirming the synovial sarcoma diagnosis.

TABLE 9.3. Common sarcoma specific fusion transcripts detected by RT-PCR.

	Fusion transcripts
Alveolar rhabdomyosarcoma	PAX3/FKHR, PAX7/FKHR
DSRCT	EWS/WT1
Ewing/PNET	EWS/FLI1, EWS/ERG, EWS/ETV1, EWS/ EIAF, and EWS/FEV
Synovial sarcoma	SSX1/SYT, SSX2/SYT, and SSX4/SYT

except in anaplastic large cell lymphoma and immunoblastic lymphoma. The key to facilitate a definitive diagnosis for lymphoma is to be able to triage the fresh specimen for flow cytometry and gene rearrangement studies when lymphoma is suspected (Fig. 9.4). Other immunohistochemical markers such as CD3, CD5, CD15, CD20, CD30, and Ki-1 are valuable in further subtyping lymphoma on cell block. Placental alkaline phosphatase (PLAP) is

TABLE 9.4. Differentiating immunostain pattern of round cell malignancy.

	CK	Synaptophysin or chromogranin or CD56 or NSE	CD45 (LCA)	PLAP	CD 117 (C-KIT)	CD 99 (MIC 2)	Desmin	Myogenin or Myo D1
Small cell carcinoma	+	+	–	–	–	–	–	–
Lymphoma	–	–	+	–	–	–	–	–
Seminoma	±	–	–	+	+	–	–	–
Ewing/PNET	±	±	–	–	–	–	–	–
DSRCT	+	+	–	–	–	±	+	–
Rhabdo myosarcoma	–	–	–	–	–	–	+	+

expressed in most seminomas. CD117 (C-KIT) is also a seminoma marker, although not specific. CK can also be occasionally positive in seminoma. Recently, there was a report that Ewing/PNET frequently expresses CK.[4,5] However, CD99 (MIC 2) is expressed in most Ewing sarcomas although is not specific. Rhabdomyosarcomas are most often positive for desmin, myogenin, or MyoD1.

For Ewing sarcoma, the hallmark cytogenetic abnormality is translocation t (11;22) and fusion transcript of EWS/FLI1 and EWS/ETS. FISH detects structural and numerical chromosomal abnormalities and works well with various cytology specimens. There are various FISH probes available for Ewing/PNET, synovial sarcoma, rhabdomyosarcoma, extraskeletal myxoid chondrosarcoma (EMC), and liposarcoma.[11–14] An example of DSRCT confirmed by cytogenetic karyotyping is illustrated in Fig. 9.5. An example of FISH study used in confirming alveolar rhabdomyosarcoma in soft tissue FNA is illustrated in Fig. 9.6.

Epithelioid Cell Morphology

Differential diagnosis includes chordoma (Fig. 9.7), EMC, epithelioid angiosarcoma, ES, epithelioid hemangioendothelioma (EH), and granular cell tumor (Table 9.5). FISH study using EWSR1 probe is useful in confirming EMC when the diagnosis is not morphologically and immunocytochemically apparent.[15]

Lipid Cell Morphology

Differential diagnosis includes lipoma, spindle cell lipoma, angiomyolipoma (AML), and liposarcoma (Table 9.6). Commonly encountered liposarcomas include atypical lipomatous tumor/well-differentiated liposarcoma, myxoid/round cell liposarcoma (Fig. 9.8), dedifferentiated liposarcoma, and pleomorphic liposarcoma. When the diagnosis is not apparent based on clinical and morphological information, FISH is useful for the differential diagnosis of liposarcomas and their cytological mimickers.[2–14] Atypical lipomatous tumor/well-differentiated liposarcoma, dedifferentiated liposarcoma and pleomorphic sarcoma frequently have

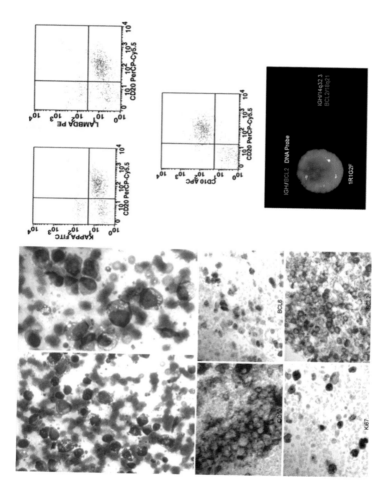

Fig. 9.4. Ancillary study in follicular lymphoma involving soft tissue. A 70-year-old female with no previous significant medical history presented with a large mesenteric soft tissue mass. A CT-guided fine needle aspiration biopsy was performed. DQ stain (x400 *upper* & x200 *lower*) reveals a cellular aspirate with a mixture of centrocytes (small cleaved cells) and centroblasts (larger noncleaved cells) in variable proportions with scant cytoplasm. Characteristic abnormal deeply folded, cleaved nucleus, "coffee bean" shape with coarse chromatin and small and inconspicuous nucleoli. Mitoses are few. Flow cytometry demonstrates a follicular B-cell lymphoma. The immunostain shows positivity with CD10, Bcl-2, and scattered Ki-67 and Bcl-6. FISH confirms the translocation of IGH and Bcl-2 genes.

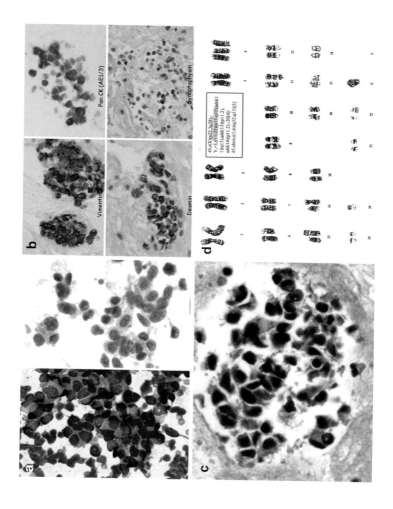

Fig. 9.5. Ancillary study in desmoplastic small round cell tumor (DSRCT). FNA from a 35-year-old man with a retroperitoneal mass. The DQ stain (x400), PAP stain (x400) and cell block (H&E stain) reveal sheets of uniformly round to oval cells. Nuclear molding is seen on cell block slides. The tumor cells are positive for vimentin, pancytokeratin (AE1/AE3), and desmin. The tumor is morphologically and immunocytologically consistent with DSRCT. Karyotyping of fresh tumor tissue confirms the diagnosis by demonstrating the characteristic translocation of chromosome 11 and 22.

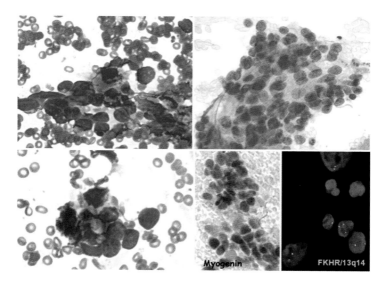

FIG. 9.6. Ancillary study in alveolar rhabdomyosarcoma. FNA from a 29-year-old female calf mass. The DQ stain (x400) and PAP stain (x400) reveal sheets of uniformly round to oval cells. Nuclear molding is seen on cell block (H&E, x400). The tumor cells are positive for vimentin and myogenin (*right lower*). The FISH study revealed FKHR/13q14 characteristics for alveolar rhabdomyosarcoma. The cytomorphology and the ancillary studies are diagnostic for alveolar rhabdomyosarcoma.

detectable MDM2–CDK4 amplification.[12,13] Myxoid/round cell liposarcoma are CHOP positive by FISH.[14] IHC can also detect MDM2 or CDK4 expression in liposarcoma.[12] Table 9.7 summarizes the sarcomas that can be confirmed by FISH testing.

Metastatic Disease Morphology

In working up bone and soft tissue tumors, metastatic disease should always be in the differential diagnosis especially for patients with prior cancer history (Table 9.8). This is best illustrated by Figs. 9.9–9.12.

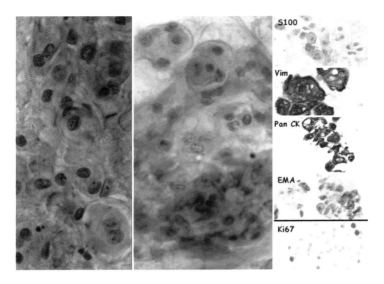

FIG. 9.7. Ancillary study in chordoma. FNA of a sacrum mass. Pap stain (*left*, x400) reveal epithelioid tumor cells in cohesive clusters and cords in a granular and fibrillary myxoid matrix. Physaliphorous cells are large tumor cells with abundant cytoplasm and conspicuous cytoplasmic vacuoles. The tumor cells are positive for S100, vimentin, pancytokerain (AE1/AE3), EMA, and focally positive for Ki-67. The cytomorphology and the ancillary studies are diagnostic for chordoma.

TABLE 9.5. Immunostain patterns of epithelioid cell malignancy.

	CK	EMA	CD31	CD34	S-100
Chordoma	+	+	−	−	−
EMC	−	−	−	−	+
Angiosarcoma	±	−	+	±	−
ES	+	+	−	+	−
EH	±	−	+	−	−
Granular cell tumor	−	−	−	−	+

In summary, immunocytochemistry and molecular testing are valuable in routine cytological diagnosis of bone and soft tissue sarcoma when they are applied in conjunction with clinical, radiological, and morphological information. With the evolution

TABLE 9.6. Differentiating immunostain pattern of lipoid malignancy.

	CD34	MDM2	CDK4	HMB45
Lipoma	–	–	–	–
Spindle cell lipoma	+	–	–	–
AML	+	–	–	+
Liposarcoma	–	+	+	–
Myxoid liposarcoma	–	–	–	–

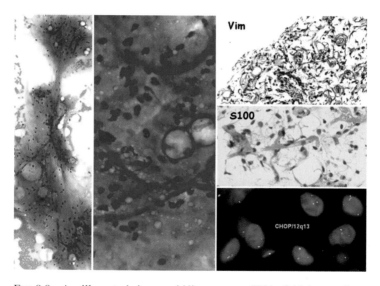

FIG. 9.8. Ancillary study in myxoid liposarcoma. FNA of thigh mass from a 30-year-old man. DQ stain (x100 *left* & x400 *right*) reveals vacuolated lipoblasts in abundant granular myxoid matrix with delicate, branching, and thin-walled vessels. The tumor cells are immunoreactive for vimentin and S-100. FISH study confirms the translocation of CHOP/12q13 genes. The cytomorphology and the ancillary studies are diagnostic of myxoid liposarcoma.

in molecular testing and the increase of minimally invasive procedures that yield decreased sample size, this multidisciplinary approach will ensure accurate diagnosis to facilitate better management of sarcoma patients.

TABLE 9.7. List of sarcomas that can be confirmed by FISH testing.

Tumor	Genes
Alveolar soft part sarcoma	ASPL, TFE3
Clear cell sarcoma	EWSR1, ATF1
Dermatofibrosarcoma protuberans	COL1A1, PDGFB
Desmoplastic small round cell tumor	EWSR1, WT1
Ewing sarcoma/primitive neutoectodermal tumor	EWSR1, FLI1
	EWSR1, ERG
	EWSR1, ETV1
	EWSR1, FEV
	EWSR1, E1AF
	EWSR1, ZSG
Extraskeletal myxoid chondrosarcoma	EWSR1, CHN
	RBP56, CHN
	CHN, TCF12
Liposarcoma, well differentiated	MDM2, CDK4
Liposarcoma, myxoid/round cell	CHOP, FUS
Low-grade fibromyxoid sarcoma	FUS, CREB3L1 or 2
Rhabdomyosarcoma, alveolar	PAX3, FKHR
	PAX7, FKHR
Synovial sarcoma	SSX1 or 2, SYT

TABLE 9.8. IHC panels that can help for tumors of unknown origin.

Lung: TTF-1, Surfactant protein A, CK7
Breast: GCDFP-15, Mamma globin, ER, PR, CK7
Prostate: PSA, PSAP, Racemase/P504S
Renal: CK, Vimentin, EMA, CD10, CA-9
Hepatocellular carcinoma: CD10, CD34, Hep Par1, CEA
Urothelial carcinoma: CK7, CK20, p63, p16, thrombomodulin
Lymphoma: CD20, CD3, Kappa, Lambda, CD45/LCA
Melanoma: S100, HMB45, Melan-A
Sarcoma: Vimentin, S100, SMA, Desmin
Small blue cell tumor: Desmin, CD99, S100, CK, Synaptophysin, CD56, CD45

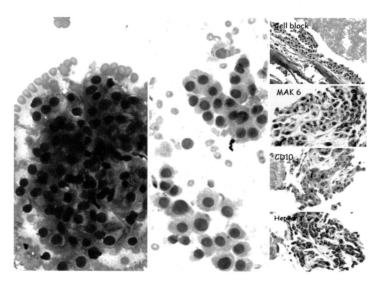

Fig. 9.9. Ancillary study in metastatic hepatocellular carcinoma. FNA of left elbow bone lesion from a 62-year-old male. DQ stain (x400) and Pap stain (x400) reveal epithelioid cells in clusters. Some cells have abundant and granular cytoplasm. Cell block (H&E, x100) reveals oncocytic tumor cells arranged in sheets. The tumor cells are positive for HepPar 1, MAK 6, and CD10, supporting the diagnosis of metastatic hepatocellular carcinoma.

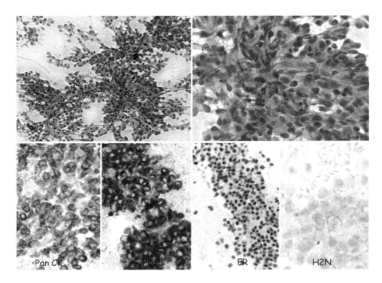

FIG. 9.10. Ancillary study in metastatic breast carcinoma. FNA of left humerus/fracture: Pap stain (x200 *left* & x400 *right*), *upper*, and immunostain study on cell block, *lower* ; from a 75-year-old female, with no history of malignancy. The patient presented with a pathological fracture of left humerus. The immunostain study on cell block (*lower*) shows positive staining for pancytokeratin (AE1/AE3), gross cystic fluid protein 15 (GCFP), estrogen receptor (ER), and negative Her2Neu (H2n), confirming a metastasis from the breast primary.

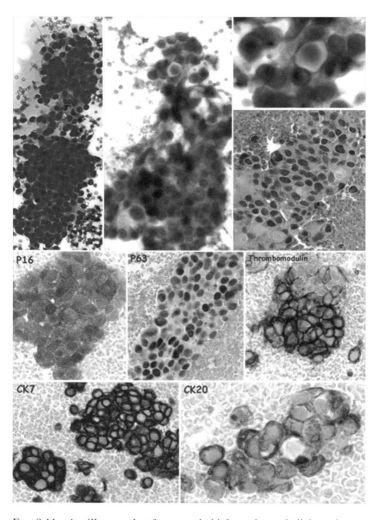

FIG. 9.11. Ancillary study of metastatic high-grade urothelial carcinoma (DQ stain, x200 *left* and Pap stain (x400 & x600) and cell block (H&E, 400), *upper*; and immunostain study on cell block, *lower*) from a 71-year-old female, with no history of malignancy, who presented with a lytic bone lesion in the L5 region. Immunostain study on cell block (*lower*) shows positive staining for CK7, CK20, p16, p63, and thrombomodulin, confirming a metastasis from the high-grade urothelial carcinoma primary.

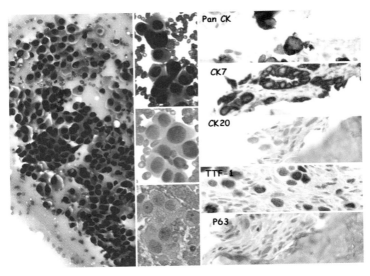

Fɪɢ. 9.12. Ancillary study of metastatic lung adenocarcinoma to the iliac bone (DQ stain, *left* x200, *upper middle* x400, Pap stain (*middle* x400), and cell block (*middle, lower* H&E, x400), *left* , and immunostain study on cell block, *right*) The patient is a 60-year-old female, with no history of malignancy, who presented with lung masses and the iliac bone lesion. Immunostain study on cell block shows positive staining for pancytokeratin (AE1/AE3), CK7; TTF-1, and negative staining for CK20 and p63, confirming a metastasis from the lung adenocarcinoma primary.

References

1. Fisher C. The comparative roles of electron microscopy and immunohistochemistry in the diagnosis of soft tissue tumors. *Histopathology*. 2006;48(1):32–41.

2. Shirazi N, Kadam V, Deodhar K, Shet T. Ultrastructure in resolving a diagnosis of poorly differentiated clear cell sarcoma of soft parts in an adolescent male. *Indian J pathol Microbiol*. 2008;51(2):280–283.

3. Guillou L, Lamoureux E, Masse S, Costa J. Alveolar soft-part sarcoma of the uterine corpus: histological, immunocytocehmical and ultrastructural study of a case. *Virchow Arch Pathol Anat Histopathol*. 1991;418(5):467–471.

4. Srivastava A, Roseberg AE, Selig M, Rubin BP, Nielsen GP. Keratin-positive Ewing's sarcoma: an ultrastructural study of 12 cases. *Int J Surg Pathol*. 2005;13(1):43–50.

5. Gu M, Antonescu CR, Guiter G, Huvos AG, Ladanyi M, Zakowski MF. Cytokeratin immunoreactivity in Ewing's sarcoma: prevalence in 50 cases confirmed by molecular diagnostic studies. *Am J Surg Pathol.* 2000;24(3):410–416.

6. Coindre JM, Pelmus M, Hostein I, Lussan C, Bui BN, Guillou L. Should molecular testing be required for diagnosing synovial sarcoma? A prospective study of 204 cases. *Cancer.* 2003;98(12):2700–2707.

7. Kilpatrick SE, Teot LA, Stanley MW, Ward WG, Savage PD, Geisinger KR. Fine-needle aspiration biopsy of synovial sarcoma: a cytomorphologic analysis of primary, recurrent, and metastatic tumors. *Am J Clin Diagn Cytopathol.* 1999;20(1):6–9.

8. Molenaar WM, van den Berg E, Dolfin AC, Zorgdrager H, Hoekstra HJ. Cytogenetic of fine needle aspiration biopsies of sarcoma. *Cancer Genet Cytogenet.* 1995;84(1):27–31.

9. Nilsson G, Wang M, Weide J, et al. Reverse transcriptase polymerase chain reaction on fine needle aspirates for rapid detection of translocations in synovial sarcoma. *Acta Cytol.* 1998;42(6):1317–1324.

10. Du CY, Shi YQ, Zhou Y, Fu H, Zhao GF. Status and clinical analysis of c-kit and PDGFR mutations in the gastrointestinal stromal tumors. *Zhonghua Wei Chang Wai Ke Za Zhi.* 2008;11(4):371–375.

11. Lazar A, Abruzzo LV, Pollock RE, Lee S, Czeniak B. Molecular diagnosis of sarcoma. Chromosomal translocations in sarcomas. *Arch Pathol Lab Med.* 2006;130:1200–1207.

12. Sirvent N, Coirdre JM, Maire G, et al. Detection of MDM2-CDK4 amplification by fluorescence in situ hybridization in 200 paraffin-embedded tumor samples: utility in diagnosing adipocytic lesions and comparison with immunohistochemistry and real-time PCR. *Am J Surg Pathol.* 2007;31(10):1476–1489.

13. Shimada S, Ishizawa T, Ishizawa K, Matsumura T, Hasegawa T, Hirose T. The value of MDM2 and CDK4 amplifiation levels using real-time polymerase chain reaction for the differential diagnosis of liposarcomas and their histologic mimickers. *Hum Pathol.* 2006;37(9):1123–1129.

14. Sugita S, Seki K, Yolozawa K, et al. Analysis of CHOP rearrangement in pleomorphic liposarcomas using fluorescence in situ hybridization. *Cancer Sci.* 2009;100(1):82–87.

15. Downs-Kelly E, Goldblum JR, Patel RM, et al. The utility of fluorescence in situ hybridization (FISH) in the diagnosis of myxoid soft tissue neoplasms. *Am J Surg Pathol.* 2008;32(1):8–13.

Index

Printed in the United States of America